# Singing in the Pain:

# My Dance with Chronic Illness

I would like to dedicate this book to my friends and family, who have been so extraordinary to me throughout this journey. I would also like to dedicate this to all of you who struggle with any sort of chronic illness or pain; We are a special breed.

# Preface

I first would like to thank you for picking up this book in whatever form that you did. It means a lot to me. This book is self- written, self- edited, and self- published, so I am sure that there may be grammar mistakes and errors. Consider this just part of the ambiance of the book! I have written about a few aspects. First, I will dive into my journey into chronic pain: how it started, what I went through, and my thoughts while dealing with everything that went on in my life over these last 8 years. You will hear directly from several people that I saw for treatments, explain just what it is that they do, how it helped me and how it may help you. The difference is that these are treatments that you may not have heard of before, and the reason I wanted to include them in this book is to shed a light on them, and make more people aware of them.

The second part of the book I will write about what I learned throughout this whole process, not only about myself, but about life in general. I will try to explain the strategies that I have incorporated to try to get the most out of my life while dealing with chronic pain and illness - strategies that have helped the mental side of what I have gone through. Lastly, I thought it was important to include a part of the book with the thoughts of those who have been through this journey with me: friends and family. This includes what they have been through, and what they have learned, directly in their own words. I have also included a question and answer segment at the very end, answering some of the most common questions people have asked me that I was not able to cover in the book.

I also want to mention that you do not need to be living with chronic pain or illness to read, relate, or learn from this book. I have tried to write this for everybody. I have tried to explain things in the simplest way that I can. I am not looking for pity, or sympathy. I wanted to just write about my experience in the hopes that it may help others, and in the hopes that it will raise awareness about what people like me go through. I have included my contact information on the last page of the book, should you want to get in touch for any reason. I think that many people go through some hard times in their life, and this is just the story of mine. So, grab an adult beverage (or three), your favourite blanket, and turn your phone to silent. Hope you enjoy!

<u>PART 1: The Journey</u>

## Chapter 1: Calm Before the Storm (1989-2012)

Since my journey into the chronic pain world, a world like living through beer goggles, does not start until my early 20s; I thought I might give a bit of a backstory about myself. I think it is important to establish who I was - a protagonist in this adventure - before my world got turned upside down. My life before pain was largely uneventful, but perhaps you would like to get to know who I was before this all started.

My father, a noble henchman, and my mother, a poor dairy farmer……oh wait wrong story. My life growing up was not anything too crazy. I grew up in a middle-class household and lived in Calgary all my life.

Much of my childhood was ordinary. I loved to play sports, any sports that involved a ball really. I played in soccer and baseball leagues, and many other sports just with friends or with my dad. As a family we went on a few vacations a year, frequently visiting the west coast of Canada and the United States. I had many hobbies in my early childhood which included: collecting pogs, rocks, hockey and baseball cards, lego, and all the usual childhood crazes of the 90s - I think I still hear my neighbor

Sarah playing Spice Girls and Backstreet Boys on her portable boom box even today.

I was a decent student in school. I got good marks, and always of course looked forward to gym class the most.

I never had any sort of illness, broken bones, or medical issues growing up, other than a bunch of ear infections at about the age of 5 that went away.

The biggest events to happen to me growing up involved 3 concussions in the span of 10 months when I was 11. As well, very bad bullying that went on for years in middle school. These issues will come up later in the book, so I will not dive into them right now.

High school was generally a good time, and I met a lot of people that I remain friends with today. The transition from high school into the real world was a bit of a shocker. I felt a lot of pressure to go to university, but I had no idea what to take. I had many interests - many things that I was good at - but nothing came to mind in terms of a career to have for the next 40 years. I switched from majoring in Radio and Television Broadcasting, to Sport and Rec Business and Entrepreneurship, and finally to Criminal Justice where I found my home.

An incident that perhaps shaped my future happened at a local night club when I was 19. Being the smart, well educated man that I was, I thought it would be a good idea to try and break up a shoving match between a few of my friends and another group of people. While attempting to intervene I was met with a one punch TKO to the face. I must have been unconscious for around 5 minutes, and when I woke up, I was on the side of the street. I was later told that I was carried out by a bouncer. I did not think anything of the incident, as afterwards, I had no symptoms other than a huge welt and bruise on the left side of my face. I even got a day off work because of it, bonus! I continued with my life, of course going back to this same club almost every weekend; The Back Alley was a part of life! Even as of this writing, we are unsure if this incident played any role in any symptoms that were to come.

Admittedly, I was not the best student in my first two years of university. I suppose I was unmotivated by school and put in the least amount of work required to get a good mark. I always did well in writing and essays, but never studied much for tests. I was more concerned about going out and having a good time with my friends than about what tests or assignments I had coming up. Things changed in my third year of university and I cannot pinpoint exactly what it was that made me more engaged. Maybe a little more maturity, perhaps getting tired of the drinking and club scene, and most of all I think I wanted to see just what would happen when I put my full effort into something. Things paid off and I started to do very well in school, which in turn boosted my overall confidence in myself. At the time, as well, I had several great close relationships, and it was some of the best times of my life. I was happy, I had a promising future, and things were looking great for the rest of my life.

<u>Chapter 2:</u>

## Entering the Abyss (2012-13)


Of course, this is when my journey into the 4<sup>th</sup> dimension - also known as chronic pain and illness - started. At the time, it was the beginning of 2012, and I was 22 years old. We were all saddened that the Jersey Shore would be airing its last episodes (or so we thought), and according to the Mayans, we only had until December before Doomsday would take us all. I was in the fourth year of my Criminal Justice degree, but it was at the same time, that I just started to feel not right. It was very subtle, and to me back then, not a big deal. For example, I would be with a friend slaying n00bs in Halo the video game, when out of nowhere I would suddenly become very dizzy and lightheaded. No big deal I thought, it is just one of those things that will go away in time. Initially I thought it could be food related and therefore made a few changes to my diet to see if these episodes would go away.

During the summer of 2012, these incidents became more frequent, but still not to the point that it was affecting my life in anyway; it was just a minor nuisance. I had gone to the family doctor and he did not seem concerned, so why should I? The very first episode of severe vertigo I had was after celebrating my mom's birthday at The Keg. Suddenly after dinner while walking in the parking lot, everything started spinning. This was the craziest stampede ride that I had ever been on! I laid on the pavement after an attack that lasted about 5 minutes, wondering what the heck just happened. My parents assumed that "hey, maybe this kid has a shellfish allergy", as I had just downed a dozen (okay maybe more) of shrimp at dinner time. Damn I thought, what am I going to do, I love shrimp!

For anyone that has not experienced vertigo, it is an experience that is hard to describe. The room can constantly spin, your balance is quite off, and often, you will experience severe nausea. It is a similar feeling of going on an intense rollercoaster, and the feeling you have after, but multiplied by 100. A close relative of vertigo is dizziness, but anyone that has had vertigo can tell you, it is much scarier and way more intense.

It was around this time as well - summer/fall of 2012 - when I noticed a few other changes. I was running severely low on energy. At the time I was working at a local grocery store in the produce section. Glamorous I know, but the ladies really dig it if you can pick out a good melon. My usual shifts were normally in the 7-hour range, and during the summer, I would work early mornings, and around 30 hours a week. For some reason, I could not work the usual amount I was used to working. I reduced my hours and thought, "it's okay I will feel better soon". This did not happen, as the symptoms only became more frequent and severe.

During winter break of 2012, I took a trip to Cancun for New Year's Eve with some friends. Suppose to be the time of your life, right? Again, I was left with a thirst for energy, feeling completely out of it and just not myself the whole time. One night I woke up with severe vertigo and stumbled my way into the bathroom. The frequency and severity of the vertigo I was having was increasing month by month, and this was the worst one yet. I was freaking out as I lay on the bathroom floor. It was the first time I legitimately thought I was going to die, as the room was spinning for hours, and it was hard to get a grasp on reality. It was hard to understand just what was happening. My heart was racing a million miles an hour and I could barely crawl to the bathtub to let water run down my face. I had troubles breathing, and counted by the minutes, hoping that it would end. Great, I thought, being sent home in a casket from Mexico will be my legacy. I thought of waking my friend for help, but she had long passed out from a day's worth of drinking. Hours later, the sun rose, and the vertigo had thankfully left. I went to breakfast and passed off to my friends that I just had a bad hangover, to account for me feeling unwell - even though I had hardly drunk anything all trip.

During this trip I noticed a bunch of other unusual things that were going on. Alcohol and I have never been that great of friends, but now I could barely have a drink or two before feeling not right and out of it. One drink felt like 10. As well I noticed that I was having a hard time just keeping up in a conversation. Words seemed hard to formulate, and it seemed hard to just compute thoughts when my friends were talking to me. I as well became scared of the vertigo I had just experienced and was afraid every night that I went to bed, that it would come back.

As we progress into 2013, surviving the Mayan apocalypse, as we had survived Y2K many years prior, things were still getting worse. Around springtime I was all set to do my practicum for school, at a local domestic violence probation office. I was getting some big boy clothes with a friend at Moores, thinking, how am I going to finish this practicum with all these symptoms happening, I must go to the doctor again. After a scintillating conversation with him, he concluded that I was just having anxiety and prescribed me anti-depressants. Well, of course I had anxiety, who would not if you were having attacks of vertigo, and just not feeling like yourself. I decided okay, I will give these a try and maybe it will help. I wanted so badly to finish my practicum, get that job experience, learn, and form relationships within the field.

I loved my time working at the probation office, but, as I tried to press on with what I was going through, my body was fighting back, and winning. Every morning I would take the bus into downtown, and there were a few occasions where I had to get off a few stops early because I would become very sick. The poor lady at the Subway near my office probably was wondering why I was running full speed into the bathroom first thing most mornings.

Even doing my job was so difficult, and I could barely concentrate. I remember one instance where I was hearing Eminem play over the speaker system in my office. Wow, this is wicked but weird that they would play Eminem. Many people came in and out of my office over the next hour or so before my boss came over and told me to shut my IPod off. Eminem was not being played over the speaker system; it was coming from my headphone speakers in my pocket. Like in Mexico, I was having a hard time formulating words and thoughts, which of course was a critical aspect of my job since I was interacting with offenders in person and over the phone all day. When I tried to write reports, I could barely type out anything. I just could not think properly. I felt very bad and that I was not only letting myself down, but also work. This was my chance to shine, show my skills, and hopefully get hired on after, or at least get a good reference. I was getting very upset because I was not myself. There were multiple instances where I had to leave work early or had to call in sick. Finally, I had to make the decision that I could not do the work and had to drop out. It was such a sinking feeling, but I knew something was not right, and I thought maybe having some time off and resting would make things better. I had a good relationship with my advisor at school, and it was a relief to me that she understood and had sympathy to what I was going through. As well she let me know I could return whenever I was ready.

<u>Chapter 3:</u>

## Oh Boy, It Gets Intense (2013-14)

The intense part of the journey started at the end of May 2013. I had bought tickets to see Mick Foley, or "Mankind" of WWE wrestling, perform stand-up comedy. Who does this guy think he is? I want to watch him bomb on stage. Unfortunately, I never made it, as I was feeling very unwell. The next morning, I woke up, and all hell had broken loose. As I got up from bed, expecting to enjoy a nice bowl of apple cinnamon cheerio's, I was greeted instead with the world spinning, the floor moving, the walls melting; and this was no fun house mirror! Something was wrong. Instead of lasting a few minutes or hours like previous episodes of vertigo, this did not go away. I went to an urgent care center a few times, but it seemed it was not taken seriously. 'Oh, you just have the flu' he said, 'and you are probably dehydrated. Go home and rest.'

As I watched French Open Tennis that weekend, watching Rafael Nadal, and his damned good looks, I thought, this was no flu. I could not concentrate on the TV, I could not think straight, and everything was continuing to shift and spin. It was hard to even keep my eyes open. Everybody, including myself, thought it was no big deal and that things would end soon. Later that month I tried to go back to my job in produce, but on my first shift back, the floors seemed to be on an angle, and I couldn't even lift up a box without falling over. I quickly left and ended up taking a leave of absence. The customers would not be getting their apples from me for a little while.

These symptoms continued every day for the summer of 2013. I did my own research about vertigo online and saw that there was a specialist at a nearby hospital. This was my ticket I thought. For some odd reason, my doctor seemed hesitant to refer me there. "Oh" he said, "your anxiety must just be getting worse to account for your symptoms, but I guess I can refer you". My days were mostly filled with lying around the house and watching as many episodes of Third Rock from the Sun as I could.  I could barely walk, could not drive, and I did not want most of my friends to see me in this condition. What would they think if I told them what was going on? Would they not take me seriously and laugh just like everyone else seemed to? I looked fine on the outside, which made it difficult for anyone to know that there was something wrong.

I remember forcing myself out for dinner with a friend, at a fancy Asian fusion restaurant. Sparkling bottled water, flower petals dawning the table, and entrees that ran into the $40 dollar range. We talked, and the word cancer came up. I knew what I was going through was serious, and when you do not know what's wrong, that word comes to mind. I remember being on the verge of tears as I chowed down on my $30 mango, papaya shrimp salad. I will be damned if I cannot at least enjoy some shrimp!

The next few months remained uneventful. My doctor deemed my case as not urgent, so I had to wait 6 months to get in to see the vertigo specialist. Meanwhile I was trying to continue as if life was normal. I forced myself back to work in produce, and even entered what I hoped would be the last year of university. However new symptoms were popping up, seemingly, weekly. I was now dealing with very severe nausea all the time, the kind you feel right before you run to the porcelain god.  As well, I started having constant pain in what felt like my ears, but it was more like the kind of pain you get when you go up in an airplane, and your ears don't pop, times about 100. I constantly had a headache as well. I proceeded to try and find anything to help me and my symptoms, from edible marijuana, to various types of drugs prescribed by my doctor, but nothing seemed to work. I even went to the eye doctor and got the BIGGEST, nerdiest, pair of glasses they had to see if they would help, but it was to no avail. When the prescription drugs did not work, I turned to natural remedies at a health food store, but they just proved to be a waste of money. School unsurprisingly, proved to be very difficult. Sitting in a huge classroom with other students, while dealing with all these symptoms was unsettling to say the least. I was able to get a medical exemption, and thankfully was able to finish most of the work and tests at home.

Months later finally the day of the big visit to the specialist arrived and I figured I was going to be saved. Currently, it was January 2014. I was hooked up to several electrodes, probably looking something like a Frankenstein creation. They were testing several nerves to see if and how well they were working. Water was plunged into my ears, creating a pressure that felt like you had stayed down in the deep end too long at the local swimming pool. A few eye tests were done as well. The conclusion from the specialist was that I had vestibular nerve damage. The vestibular nerve plays several functions, mainly balance and coordination. Damage to this nerve causes attacks of vertigo, nausea/vomiting, and an inability to maintain balance and coordination. Success! I had a diagnosis! Okay doc, how do we fix this so I can get back to my life? Her response made my heart drop. 'Well,' she said, 'sometimes the nerve can regenerate itself, but can take a number of years. Sometimes the nerve cannot regenerate itself, and the brain, over a long period of time, again years, must adapt. There is no magical cure for this. Some people suffer from it their whole lives, and if you've already had symptoms for this long, you may have what is called Meniere's disease, a disorder of the inner ear which causes all the symptoms that you have.'

Well, this was not the answer I was looking for, and we had not even finished the appointment yet. 'I am concerned,' she continued, 'that you have as well, a number of other symptoms that aren't associated with one that has vestibular nerve damage.' She did a quick physical, after which she said, 'do you realize that your lower jaw is severely displaced? You need to see your dentist.' I had no idea about my jaw, and after the appointment I was mentally exhausted. Walking out of the room, and watching my mom break down into tears after I told her the results really made the whole situation real to me. My mom then told me that she did not know if I legitimately had something wrong with me, because she thought, well, you've been to a bunch of doctors and they seemed to think it was all mental, and you had nothing wrong, so I believed them.

Coming home that night I had a lot to think about. It was devastating to hear the news from the specialist, but not only that, to hear that my own mom, for a long period of time, had doubts about what was going on with me. I have always prided myself in being an honest person, and while I tend to have a big mouth, and maybe gossip more than I should, I never lie about things, and am not one to over exaggerate something. I was wondering, if my own mom had doubts about there being something medically wrong with me, what did other people think? Along with that, I asked myself, how can I keep going if I am going to have to deal with these symptoms for a much longer period? I had become mentally, physically, and just overall drained. My body was in such a state of stress that my hair was falling out - thankfully not permanently. I was riddled with anxious thoughts, every day, and all the time. Anxious about everything. About going to work, about hanging out with friends, about going anywhere, or doing anything. My symptoms had left me a shell of my former self, on the inside. On the outside I was still able to pass off as the same old laid-back person.

When the world is constantly spinning, month after month, it becomes a scary place. It almost seemed like I was in an alternate reality, it almost seemed like it was not real life anymore – there was a glitch in the Matrix, and I could not fix it. How could someone feel this bad? Making it through the day was an accomplishment to me. I no longer wanted to hang out with my friends as I could barely hold a conversation. At this time, I could no longer continue school, even though I only had two classes left to finish my degree. I could not read pages in a book, as everything was blurry and moving. I could not concentrate at all on anything. I could not play sports or even walk for more than a few minutes, as I could barely stay upright on my feet. Everything that I loved to do was seemingly gone.

I tried to maintain a positive outlook and made sure that I could do everything that I could do physically. I kept a few shifts a week at work and was surprisingly still able to work out at the gym. After seeing my dentist, he had the same conclusion as the vertigo specialist, but he did not have any expertise in the jaw, so he sent me to a jaw specialist. But again, I had to wait months.

In May 2014 I saw this specialist, and the findings were quite eye opening. He found a fracture in my jaw on the left side, but it had healed. As well he noted that my jaw was severely shifted and dislocated to one side of my face. He made a comment that the only time he has ever seen this before is someone who has had major trauma to their face, such as a car accident. We went over my prior history and tried to think of how this could have happened, but the only thing that came to mind was the punch to the face in the night club years prior. He could not say for sure if that had anything to do with how my jaw was today. After many appointments and procedures, a splint was made, that was supposed to gradually shift my jaw back into place. I had nice big monkey cheeks afterwards. I felt a sense of optimism that this was finally going to be the thing to help me.

However the pain I was having in my jaw, and in my head only got worse and was beginning to be very severe, while at the same time, dealing with all the other symptoms I had been going through. One new thing I was experiencing frequently was depersonalization, or derealization. In a nutshell this is basically when things do not seem real or seem dream-like. Feelings of detachment from oneself, sort of like you are playing yourself in a video game. As lax as this definition is, depersonalization is incredibly terrifying to experience. My fight or flight response was super high, daily, and nonstop, which, with my symptoms I figured was contributing to this feeling.

 Now that I had medical proof that I indeed had nerve damage, as well as a severely dislocated jaw, I was finally able to try out several other medications. Soon after though, I had started to experience severe pain in my urethra, as well as my prostate. It was an intense pain, and when it was at its worst, I could not even sit down. After several images, as well as having a camera up my urethra, it was found that I had large cysts that were causing the issue. It was later determined after many months of severe pain that some of the medications I had been using were causing the issue. When I got off the medication, the pain thankfully disappeared. And yes, the camera up the urethra was as pleasant as it sounds!

It was now summer of 2014, and i was just playing the waiting game. Waiting for the nerve damage to heal, waiting for the splint to move my jaw in the right direction, waiting for my symptoms to get better. But as the months and months passed, nothing got better. I played countless games of backgammon and crib with my dad; I needed something, anything, to pass the time. Most of my days were still spent on the couch...My television show of choice this summer was Night Court.

A year went by with no results but was continuously told by my specialists and doctors to be patient. I wanted to scream and yell at them, and tell them just what kind of hell I was living in. Obviously, the severity of my symptoms was not getting through to them. I always came to my appointments smiling, making jokes, and laughing, because that is just who I am. I am not going to let anything define me or bring me down. I now realize perhaps when explaining my symptoms to doctors and specialists, that, because I was smiling and laughing with them, and looked fine on the outside, I was not taken as seriously as I should have.

<u>Chapter 4:</u>

## What Else Could Go Wrong? (2015-16)

Throughout the beginning of 2015, my sleeps were increasingly getting worse, and I would wake up multiple times a night choking, gasping for air, and barely able to breathe. I decided to get a private sleep study done to figure out exactly what was going on. The sleep doctors made the diagnosis of moderate sleep apnea, caused by my jaw blocking part of my airway. I was having around 20-25 episodes an hour of waking up from lack of oxygen. I rented a CPAP machine for a few months, thinking it would cure my problem, and perhaps if I had a better sleep, I would be able to deal with my pain and symptoms better. But unfortunately, the machine did not help me...other than looking super sexy for the girls.

The summer of 2015 turned out to be not a bad summer at all. The symptoms that I had associated with vertigo, were less, and the pain, although still very much there, seemed more manageable. I deem some of this success to a new therapist that I was seeing. She did craniosacral work, and I will explain this in a bit more detail in a later chapter. As the summer went on, I was able to even pick up more shifts at work and felt like I was making progress on several fronts. And, for the first time in almost two years, I had an appetite. This did a great deal for me mentally, as for years now, it felt like I was stuck in a rut, making no progress. I was finally starting to enjoy activities and felt more like myself. I was even able to enjoy half a dozen or so rounds of golf, and spent many nights at the driving range, as it was one activity, I could do that did not induce any symptoms.

I also greatly focused on going to the gym. It was a life saver to me, as I could release all the pent-up anger, I had that was associated with what was going on with me. It was also cool to see how much progress that I was making, and it gave me something else to focus on other than my medical issues. I spent many nights with friends like old times, enjoying the moment, instead of suffering through it. I did watch less television this summer, but my show of choice was catching up on all the seasons and episodes of Breaking Bad.

Unfortunately, the progress I was making changed, when one day at work in October 2015, while lifting a heavy box, I felt several pops and burning sensations in my neck, down my traps and into my shoulder. I knew something was very wrong. It took a long time to get a proper idea of what exactly I had happened, and what was injured. When it was all said and done, they found that I had torn a muscle in my left shoulder, tore my left trap, and partially tore several ligaments in my neck and upper back.

It was realized, almost a year later that the tears were caused because, my jaw being greatly out of place, was putting a great amount of strain on my neck muscles. This strain was causing the neck muscles, and those muscles surrounding the neck to be very weak and susceptible to injury. If I had not injured it at work, it was likely that I would have at the gym or doing some other activity. I had to wear a neck brace, and it was hilarious to me that I received more sympathy while wearing that for a week, than I had the prior 2 years combined.

Obviously at this time I was left unable to work, and so began the journey of physiotherapy therapy to try and get back to full strength. A few months went by though, and nothing had healed. What was going on? My jaw was not getting any better or moving into a better place, and now, the injuries I sustained were not healing at all. It was January 2016 when I decided to get another opinion on my jaw. I trusted the specialist I was seeing, as everyone recommended him, and he seemed like the only true jaw specialist in my city, but, I was literally seeing no results at all, and he was giving me no ideas about how to proceed.

I got a few different opinions from dentists that also dealt with the jaw, and they had come to the same conclusion that my jaw was still severely shifted and dislocated. However, these dentists had a different method of making a splint, one that used sensors and electrodes to properly map out the best position of the jaw. Once that position was found, a mould would be made for a brace, or splint, that, like the first splint I had, was supposed to shift my jaw into its correct place. Plus, on the bright side, with their sensory equipment, I had finally found a good Halloween costume for the upcoming year.

Along with the new splint, I had a few tongue surgeries that were supposed to aid in setting my jaw in the right place. It was found at this time, that I had severe tongue tie, where I could barely push my tongue out of my mouth, and as well I couldn't rest my tongue on the top of my mouth – the palate. It was thought that this could be part of the reason that my jaw was not getting better. The tongue being able to rest at the top of the palate aids in stabilizing your jaw into a comfortable resting position. Parts of my tongue were lasered off, and I can still taste and smell what that was like, much the same as burnt hair. A beautiful aroma that should be bottled and sold in stores. A new Calvin Klein cologne perhaps.

What followed once the new splint was made and the tongue surgeries was possibly the worst set of months in a row, that I could possibly imagine someone going through. Immediately I felt my jaw starting to shift after the new splint was inserted in. However, instead of all my symptoms getting better, they got much worse. The pain started to become overwhelming again, and my vertigo came back. Combined with the injuries I still had to my neck; it was a very overwhelming situation. This time the vertigo was much more severe than it had ever been in the past. One night while watching TV. it became so intense that I started freaking out. It was lasting hours and hours, so severe to where I could not even see my hand in front of me, it was just a blur. I tried to crawl around the house to stay grounded, as sometimes just laying down made the vertigo worse. It was getting to the point where I was puking and dry heaving dozens of times, and I was having troubles breathing. Finally, my parents had to call an ambulance because it felt as though I was dying. I was in so much pain, and the vertigo was so bad, that I was having an out of body experience. It is hard to explain the sheer terror that I felt, as I was loaded into the back of the ambulance, headed for the hospital. I prayed that there was something that they could do for me.

Unfortunately, there was not. At this point I had literally tried dozens of medications, mostly for pain. However, I found I felt better taking no medications at all, as I seemed to have bad side effects, and it made the nausea I had, much worse.

For vertigo, there is not any specific medication that you can take. There is one medication, that will dilate your ear canal, but this is only effective if your vertigo is caused by water in your ears, as the dilation of the ear canal is supposed to drain the water out. While at the hospital I was given a few options for pain, such as morphine, but I feared that it would make me feel much sicker. There was nothing that the doctors could do, other than heavily sedate me with sedatives, and wait for the vertigo to die down.

Over the next month, the severity continued and there was three more instances where I went to the hospital. Again, there was nothing that they could do, except offer me different cocktails of drugs. One of the times ketamine was offered. Could you imagine having severe vertigo, and then being dissociated from your own body, as that is what ketamine does. I did not want to find out what that felt like! The only good thing about going to the hospital was obviously the fashion. I felt the blue scrubs really brought out the color in my eyes! Unfortunately, they would not let me bring a pair home.

Both of my parents were saints during this period of distress. I relied on them heavily just to make it through the day, just to distract me, talk to me and comfort. They would take me on car rides to the local baseball diamond, and I would watch, usually from the car, young kids playing the game I loved and played for 20 years, on the same diamond. They would take me on drives all over the city, visiting neighborhoods we either had never been to, or had not been in awhile. Often these were rich neighborhoods with gigantic houses, and we would guess how much they would pay their gardener. They took me on walks, even though I could barely last 5 minutes. They would drive me to all my appointments, or wherever I needed to go.  Every day we would play countless games of backgammon, crib, and other card games.

Most days they would stay up past their usual bedtime, and watch late night comedies with me, or sports highlights, just to make sure I was alright. I used to wake up in the middle of the night puking, and the world spinning, and they were there for a hug, or to sit with me until the sun rose, or to offer their room.

<u>Chapter 5:</u>

## Hospitalization (2016)

It was now April 2016, and my body, and mind, was beginning to feel the effects of the trauma that I was going through. I quickly lost 40 pounds, as I was continuing to throw up, and dry heave, daily. I could barely sleep, and it was hard to think rationally. I was deadly terrified every day, that a severe episode of vertigo would happen, and I would end up right back at the hospital. At this point I knew the hospital would not help, but in my mind, it was a safe place. Finally, one day, early in May, I finally had enough of what had been going on. No one was helping, not my specialists, not my doctors, and not anybody at the emergency room. Nobody really knew what to do. The vertigo was most likely being caused by my jaw shifting because of the splint, but it must have been greatly affecting the nerves in my face, as well as my inner ear.  Normally, when someone gets a splint, they are told that it will take a couple months, maybe 6 for their jaw to get back in the right position. Because my case was so severe, the new specialist I was seeing was unsure of the timeline, or even what would happen, because she had never seen something like this.

I made the decision to yet again, head back to the emergency room, but this time, instead of focusing on telling them all of the physical things that was wrong with me, I was going to tell them how the physical things were affecting me mentally. At this point, I was very depressed. It was a struggle every minute of every day, and I did not want to go through it anymore. I had been going through this for 3 years already, and now it was much worse than ever before. There were so many times throughout the previous few years where I had hope, and where it looked like I was turning the corner. But now, I had run out of hope. I truly did not want to live anymore. I did not even look in the mirror for several weeks; I did not want to see my own face, which, at this point, was very shrunken in. Many days, I did not have the energy to even brush my teeth, or to have a shower. My body and mind were so traumatized, and scared, that I began to shake, and convulse a lot of the time. In my mind, at this time, I knew that I wanted to live, there was so many things that I loved, enjoyed doing, and that made me happy. It just felt that getting better was so far out of reach, and that I would never get there.

As well, there was my family. Every time I thought of them during this time, I started to cry. I cried because they were suffering too. I could see it in their faces. I did not want them to go through this; they did not deserve to suffer along with me. They had done everything to help me in the previous 3 years, everything that you can imagine, and everything that you can think of. They were there for me, through all the days where I cried myself to sleep, the nights spent at the hospital, driving me to all the appointments when I wasn't able to myself, and just spending time with me trying to get my mind off of what I was going through.

So, I made the decision to go in, and tell the nurses in the emergency room, all the stuff I was going through mentally as well. I figured I might be taken more seriously this time, and I was. The decision was made to hospitalize me. The first day I was in the hospital, I did not have my own room, it was just a sort of makeshift room because they had run out of beds. It was a very long day as I had come to the hospital early in the morning, and I was sitting and laying down in this room for over 12 hours. I would have a nurse come in and check on my vitals every once in awhile, but that was all the contact I had with anyone. Because they did not have a room for me, they were not sure if I would be staying at the hospital I was at, or if I were going to be transferred to another hospital across town.

I remember this time was very uneasy as I did not know what was going to happen with me, where I was going to stay, or what the next while had in store for me. Being in this little room for so long was very isolating, as I was all by myself with nothing to do, no TV, just a room with a bed, being hooked up and checked for vitals. I had a lot of time to think about things and wondering if this was the right thing to do. Other then when they told me they were going to hospitalize me; they did not really tell me much else. They did not say here is what we are going to do, here is our plan, this is how long you are going to be here for. So, there was a lot of unknown. I had no idea what was in store for me, like kinder egg surprise, except this time there was no toy.

It was quite late at night, maybe around 11pm when someone came in and said that they had a bed for me finally, and I was able to stay at this hospital. They took me in a wheelchair up to my floor and showed me around the area of which I was going to be staying. There was a tiny common room with a couple of TVs, a couple of couches, a shelf with a lot of books and board games, and little kitchen with a fridge and sink and few dining tables with chairs. There was an oddly out of place treadmill right beside the kitchen, and then two long corridors of rooms, and that was basically it. I was showed to my room which was quite small, but thankfully initially I did not have to share it with anyone. Just a hospital bed, and a bathroom and that was it.

The nurse let me know someone would be by in the morning to talk with me and left me alone to sleep for the night. Of course, I could not sleep though. So many thoughts were racing through my head. I ended up pacing around my room, my mind seemingly going a hundred miles an hour. Every time I tried to sleep, I could not as I could hear every little sound. Someone puking a few rooms down, nurses walking up and down the halls, monitors in other rooms beeping, the loud sounds of the furnace that would come on every 30 minutes. I suddenly realized that I was all alone. I did not have my mom and dad to rely on like I had so heavily for the last few months. I knew that for the next little while I would only see them during visiting hours, and that it was basically going to be me on my own.

I was awoken startlingly at 8am, which was breakfast time, and some patients in nearby rooms gathered in a common area to eat. You could eat in your room, but it seemed like not many people wanted to. Looking down at my breakfast I could not fathom eating anything, as it all looked so bleak and unappetizing. They had given me cream of wheat. I still do this day do not know what exactly it is. A liquid? A solid? Something in-between surely. All I was able to have was an orange juice. I remember trying to put my tray back into the cart, but because I was shaking so badly from my symptoms, I was not able to put it in the slot, and had to have another patient do it for me. I had a visit with a nurse who informed me that there were no activities or doctors on staff during the weekend, and no testing as well, so I was free to do whatever I wanted with my time. While talking with the nurse, I noticed my mom and dad walking down the long corridor, coming to visit me. I could not contain myself and cried probably as hard as I ever have in my life, it was very deep, and from the soul. I was so thankful to see them. They stayed for hours on end, playing cards with me, and watching the television. One of the things I remember is how uncomfortable the furniture was in the common area. I finally got my first laugh in months when I watched my dad squirm for hours trying to find a comfortable position on a couch that had little backing and that barely fit his bum.

I had such high hopes that something could be done while staying in the hospital, but again I was met with a little bit of disappointment. I was set up with a doctor for my stay to talk about medication that may help, but in my estimation, we did not talk enough. I had a long first session with her while I explained what was going on, my symptoms, what the last few years had been like, and right away she wanted to stick me on a number of medications. It was a bit disheartening as I had already tried the medications she suggested, and they did not work. But was made to feel that if I said no, then it meant that I did not want to get better.

After this first meeting, she was going to see me once a day for around 15 minutes, but I always ended up getting her student, who seemed to be in over his head, and had no empathy or understanding what I was going through. When I did not want to take the medication she suggested, the student got mad, and wondered why I was wasting everyone's time. He kept hammering home that my symptoms were caused by anxiety and depression, which was untrue. What I was dealing with was so overwhelming, and the symptoms so terrible that yes I wasn't able to do a lot, and it was hard to remain upbeat and positive,  and it that made me depressed. Not the other way around. I had so much life in me, but it was all being sucked away by what I was dealing with.

Other than discussing medications, I did not talk about much else in the short time I had every day with the doctor or the student. I was hopeful when I arrived that there may be a psychologist, or someone to regularly talk to about what I was going through and help me deal with the physical symptoms better mentally, but there was not.

The activities that they offered during the day, seemed like things just to pass the time. I am sure that the hospital is limited in what they can offer, and perhaps some people got use out of them, but for me, it was little more than a time waster. There were things such as making pita pizzas, an art class where we just drew and colored. As well a nutrition class that was very simple. White bread is bad! Sugar is bad! I almost felt like I was in a fifth-grade health class. As much as the activities were lame, it was nice to keep busy.

The other downside for me was the other patients that I was with. There were a few that I made friends with and was very thankful for their company during this time. But for the most part, everyone that was there was not in good shape and being surrounded by them for days on end, only seemed to worsen my mental state. There was a lot of crazy things that went on in or near the ward that I was staying on: security being called multiple times, fights, screaming, moaning, yelling etc. Lots of erratic behaviour. As well just a lot of people that were sick and got physically sick.

Thankfully, my parents came almost every day to visit me during visiting hours. It made it nice that the hospital was only a 5-minute drive down the road. I was so thankful for their company, as it was a nice distraction, and nice to see and talk to somebody familiar. I had many family and friends that wanted to come visit, but I was too embarrassed for them to see me in the shape I was.  I got lucky and was sent a few gift and fruit baskets, and I still keep one of the teddy bears that came with one of them, that was given to me by my aunt and uncle. I still keep by my bedside to this day as a reminder of what                     I                 went                 through.

After more testing was done on me in the few weeks I was in the hospital, I was released. The decision was made by my doctors that I needed to focus more on my mental well-being. They had realized that yes, I did have severe medical symptoms and pain, but they felt that I needed to focus more on my mental health, than I was doing. I was set up with a psychologist that would help me deal with my pain better, and as well, given a few workbooks and tools to help me. I was also set up with a neurologist to go over imaging and try out different medications and injections for pain.

<u>Chapter 6:</u>

## Post Hospitalization (2016)

It was a few weeks after leaving the hospital that I had my first visit with my psychologist. At first, I had a few reservations about seeing and talking to someone. Of course, for the last few years I seem to have not been taken seriously or dismissed by a lot of professionals. I had a fear that this would be the same thing. I as well had tried to see a psychologist a year prior, but we did not connect, and I did not pursue it further. This other psychologist was older, and very cookie cutter in her ways. It basically seemed like she had a formula, and I was just another person to plug into her algorithm of how to treat people.

I thought that this psychologist might be the same. My story was also so long, different, and a little hard to understand that It was a little scary telling everything to someone who did not know me at all. Of course, there was also the part of me that thought that I did not need to see or talk to someone because I was already very open and honest about everything with my friends and family. Looking back this was just something I told myself to give credence to the fact that I was a bit afraid of going.

Thankfully, I really seemed to connect with this psychologist right off the bat. It was almost like going to see a friend. I had the initial thoughts that she would kind of tell you what to do, and have their own opinions on how to help you with little input from myself, but it wasn't like that at all. She listened to what was going on with me. Listened to my frustrations, what my thoughts were, what my emotions were, and she was basically just a guide. She helped push me in a direction that I was already going, but with a little bit of encouragement. She offered up her support, the tools that she knew, the coping mechanisms that she thought could help me, and tailored those things to what I was going through. A lot of the coping mechanisms were things I was already aware of, but she made me see them in a different light and made them less daunting and easier to implement.

I realized quickly that I needed that outside perspective of someone that was not a friend or family member. I needed someone that did not know me, and someone that had a fresh viewpoint. She reaffirmed that what I was going through was kind of crazy, and unique, and hard, but made me feel like I wasn't insane, and that the way my mind was dealing with the physical symptoms was normal.

I think it helped that we were around the same age, and that we had the same outlook on life, and we were coming from the same place on a lot of issues, and shared many of the same values, beliefs and thoughts. The sessions were very open ended, and the floor was open to me on what I wanted to talk about, and whatever I felt like I needed to deal with.

We ended up having around 20 sessions together over the course of a year and a half, but the last few sessions ended up being mostly just talking, and less about therapy. The time had come for me to move on, she told me, "Ryan you know all the strategies, you know what needs to be done to help yourself. I don't need to give you any new information, you just have to make sure that you stay on top of everything and implement all the strategies we talked about into your everyday life."

I was surprised during the last session how sad I felt, because it felt like I was losing a friend. I remember asking, are you sure that I cannot see you one last time? I will always be thankful for the time that we shared together. She saw me at my worst, when I came into a lot of the sessions crying or started crying in the middle of a session. She saw me when I was having a good day and was talkative and happy. She gave me the confidence to continue trucking on in my journey, and a lot of skills to take on my way.

After leaving the hospital, I was also set up with a neurologist, to dive further into the symptoms, headaches, and migraines that I was having. Unfortunately, again, like most doctors, it was more of just trying to find out what medications might work for me. Since I had already tried almost every medication recommended, we decided to try both Botox, and nerve blocks for the migraines. Medically, Botox is used for migraines as in simple terms it freezes a certain muscle for 3 months, so it does not fire, and does not work. Botox consists of dozens of injections in the forehead, back of the neck, traps, side of the head, and in my case, the main jaw muscle, the massator.

Nerve blocks are injections that are right into the scalp, usually in the back of the head, and work by reducing inflammation that may be happening around a certain nerve. Like Botox, its kind of freezes the area, but only for a few days to a couple weeks per injection. I believe the main ingredient is a certain type of steroid. I tried many rounds of Botox, and many nerve blocks, but did not see any results from either, other than my microscopic wrinkles disappearing.

Sadly after a period of time, my neurologist dismissed me because there was not much else he said he could do for me. As well, after leaving the hospital, I decided to visit a NUCCA chiropractor, a specialized chiropractor that focuses on the first two vertebrae of the neck. I had read that a lot of people found relief from their vertigo, by seeing this type of chiropractor. Several x-rays were done on my neck, from many different angles, and the results, and what the chiropractor said, greatly surprised me. 'The first two vertebrae of your neck are severely twisted to one side' he said. 'Close to a 12-degree angle, which is quite severe. Most people that I see, they may have their vertebrae twisted a few degrees. I actually had the other chiropractor in the office come take a look at your x-rays, because they were so interesting.'

He went on to say that he believed this was not only the cause for some of my vertigo, but the cause to why my neck injuries, had not healed yet. He further explained, "Injury to the spine tears loose the connective tissue, ligaments and muscles responsible for maintaining posture and alignment. The result is a misalignment where the head, neck and atlas have shifted from their normal position. This causes stress and altered nerve flow to and from the brain and creates posture distortion and body imbalance as the entire spine shifts off center."

To me, this made perfect sense, as I still at this point was barely able to walk more than a few minutes, not only because of the dizziness, vertigo and the pain, but also because everything felt so out of whack all down my neck, and all down my back. Walking felt very disjointed, weird, and unnatural. I asked my chiropractor, Dr. Abreu, to do a small write up for the purposes of this book, as I found rarely anyone knew about this technique. I wanted him just to explain more in depth in case anybody was interested.

"With the use of specific x ray views, a NUCCA chiropractor measures the structural misalignments of your head and neck, calculates how to correct the misalignments with a precise formula, and then based on your misalignment, delivers a customized adjustment to the top of your neck to align your spine, restore postural balance, and improve nerve flow.

NUCCA chiropractors are trained to measure postural distortions. If you look at yourself, or a friend or family member, you may notice their head is tilted to one side, one shoulder may be lower than the other side, or one hip may be lower too. This may be a sign that there is muscle tension and stress points in their spine. Sometimes we feel them, and sometimes we have no idea. If you have any of those things, or notice them on others, it might be a good time to get your posture checked by a NUCCA chiropractor. The most common conditions that we see are people suffering from chronic conditions that are related to old injuries, or recent injuries such as a motor vehicle accident.

During the initial appointments, a NUCCA chiropractor will discuss your comprehensive health history, explain what a NUCCA chiropractor can do for you, measure your posture, assess your spine and take specific x-rays of your head and neck. These x-rays will be analyzed for misalignments, where we will review with you the findings, and give you your first adjustment. We will also recommend a care plan based off your exam and x-rays, and then take a second set of x-rays to measure the correction from the first adjustment. The subsequent visits after this are to monitor your progress, adjust you as needed, and to give advice on how to maintain your spinal correction. Results vary from individual to individual; everyone is unique. However, changes in your spinal alignment will happen with each adjustment, and over time your body will become stable with the NUCCA correction.

In terms of finding a qualified NUCCA chiropractor in your area, the most common place to search is online. You can also search NUCCA.org for a doctor near you. NUCCA chiropractors are all licensed chiropractors, and experience and credentials vary from doctor to doctor. NUCCA chiropractors may be board certified in the NUCCA technique, but to know if one will help you, it is best to schedule a consultation and ask questions regarding your health issues.

As mentioned earlier, often clients come to us with chronic, or recent injuries. Along with chiropractic care, a multidisciplinary approach may be required to get the most out of treatment, and to get your body back moving and functioning correctly. In our office we have physiotherapists, and message therapists that offer craniosacral therapy, integrated osteopathy, visceral manipulation, Bowen Therapy, lymphatic drainage, intraoral massage, Thai massage, and deep tissue massage. We work in coordination with our physiotherapists, and massage therapist."

The summer of 2016 consisted of seeing this chiropractor twice a week, along with physiotherapy, the psychologist, massage, exercises, and walking. I remember the first days of seeing Dr. Abreu, I was just out of the hospital, and still quite sick. Id have to carry around a puke bucket with me in the waiting room, and to the subsequent rooms. I needed to make the bucket into a necklace so it would always hang below me. Would have been fashionable and useful! As the months went on from treatment, my twisted vertebrae slowly started to get back into proper place, and the intensity and severity of my vertigo started to lessen. As well, my injuries to my neck, and back, also started to heal. I was also able to walk longer distances, but it felt so weird. It felt like I had to learn to walk again, as my vertebrae, and spine, must have been out of alignment for some time, and, for the previous years, I was unable to walk much at all. My neck felt like a noodle, it was very weak, and my head kept sloping to one side or the other, it was hard just keeping my head upright.

As you can imagine I was very pleased, but mentally, I was still having a rough time. Something had changed, after all those intense episodes of vertigo, and times where I thought I was going to die. I kept having nightmares every night, mostly of dying, and I would wake up in a panic, dripping with sweat. During the daytime, I would have vivid flashbacks of the times where I thought I was going to die, and the vertigo that I had at that time. The flashbacks are hard to describe. It is almost like all your senses go back to that period when you were experiencing great stress. I could see the room spinning like I was having vertigo, I could taste the puke in the back of my mouth, I could smell the smell of the hospital, and I could feel the cold metal of the gurney that I was loaded in while in the ambulance. All these things would flash back to me, and it left me in fear, and it left me shaking and in tears most of the time. After a while of this happening, it was later determined to be PTSD. How come I could not have flashbacks of roasting marshmallows by a fire, or pitching in the prairie championships in baseball? That would have been much better! The television show of choice this summer was Frasier, and of course Toronto Blue Jays baseball.

In the fall, if all that I had going on was not enough I was also diagnosed as having a breathing disorder. Because my jaw was so out of place, for so long, my body was not able to breathe properly, and it compensated for this by taking huge inhales, and short exhales. I was told that basically I was reverse hyperventilating. My jaw was back into a better place currently, but I was breathing as if my jaw was still blocking my airway. It was found that my body was taking in too much oxygen, and not expelling out enough carbon dioxide. As well, at lot of times, I would hold my breath, for minutes at a time, not realizing it. I learned as well that chronic pain can affect your breathing quite severely. Like walking, now I basically had to learn how to breathe properly again. It sounds easy, but, after many years of compensation, my body was used to breathing a certain way, and I found it very challenging to reverse this. Doing the breathing exercises, and while trying to breathe normally, it felt so foreign, that it often left me feeling very weird, and dizzy. I felt somewhat like a lab rat, where we were trying to rebuild me from scratch.

<u>Chapter 7:</u>

## Trying to Solve the Puzzle (2017)

It was great at this time that so many things that were wrong, were being treated for, or looked after. I had so many appointments that I felt like a celebrity in the chronic pain and illness world. However, I felt as though we were not still dealing with the root problem of the issue, which at this time, I thought was still the jaw. My family and I were becoming experts on local specialists in the area, and we decided at this time to head to the U of A hospital in Edmonton, where they had a dentistry team that saw unique cases. As you can imagine I was thrilled when my first "vacation" outside of the city in years was to Edmonton in the middle of winter. For those of you that are in the United States, it is like going to Wisconsin...with out the good beer and cheese. My dad and I made the 3-hour drive north, and as always, I was cautiously optimistic.

The experience was quite a full day. I filled out a few in-depth questionnaires to begin with and was shown to a room where I would be for the next few hours or so. I basically saw a team of people, one right after another. Dentists, physiotherapists, oral surgeons, orthodontists. For each one I would go through my story, go through several tests on my jaw and neck, and they looked at all the available images that they had. In the end their recommendation was major jaw surgery, and as well be on a constant dose of methadone for the pain.

Their conclusions did not surprise me, but I wanted to get more opinions from local surgeons in Calgary, if jaw surgery was the best idea. I also refused to be on methadone. On top of everything else I was going through I did not want to be on a constant dose of opiates and have to deal with those withdrawals sometime in the future. I also did not want to become addicted. I was already having troubles with staying awake and energy, with methadone I felt I would just be nothing more than a vegetable and a wobbling head, struggling to keep my eyes open. I was not able to do much still, but I savoured the moments I could.

After a few months wait, I was finally able to see a surgeon in Calgary. I learned over the years that I was taken much more seriously if I was with a parent, or a friend, as opposed to by myself. Early on all my appointments I was there alone, and that's when I always got brushed off, so over time, and because my situation was so complex, I learned it was better to have someone come with me to corroborate my story. My mom came to this specialist's appointment, and I am glad she did, because still to this day we laugh about the experience.

This surgeon was one of the most ignorant and dismissive individuals that I encountered during my journey. He flat out refused to even acknowledge surgery as an option and laughed it off. We tried to ask questions and to why his opinion was so different than the surgeons in Edmonton, but he was not really listening to us. After only seeing me for about 5 minutes, he wanted to leave, basically only saying no you do not need surgery, goodbye. I tried asking him what I should do in my situation then. Obviously, things were wrong, and something needed to be done, but what? He answered that I should try eating softer foods and to use an icepack. The appointment was then over.

As my mom and I left the appointment, we were taken back at what just happened. Other chronic illness/pain sufferers will know all too well the feeling that I had that day. To be so dismissed. To feel laughed at. To feel like I was wasting his time. And on top of that, to be given such horrendous advice as to just eat soft foods and use an ice pack. Obviously, the severity of the situation was not grasped by this surgeon, as it was not by so many before him. To me, it felt insulting, to be given that "advice". I had literally been driven almost insane by the severity of my symptoms yet was passed off like I just had a tiny ache in my jaw. Little did he know I already did have my own little rotation of ice packs of all makes and sizes, so take that!

Again, I was at a loss of what to do next. Because there was such a discrepancy in what the different surgeons said, I did not feel comfortable going through any kind of procedure. I learned from much research, that of course anything you do like surgery, is permanent, and cannot be undone. Although sucking a steak smoothie through a straw was intriguing, there was no guarantee that it would make things better, and if anything, it could make things worse.

I cannot stress enough that when you are in a situation like mine, how much time is spent researching, reading, and trying to just figure out what the hell was going on. Early on, I relied on the word of my doctors for everything. But of course, as you have read, this did not help me. I had become accustomed to, out of necessity, trying to research the best possible action to take for myself. If only I had studied this hard in high school! It was hard, because there were so many symptoms, and seemingly so many things going on at the same time. We knew the symptoms, but what was the underlying cause? Why was I feeling like this? Was it all the jaw, or was there more going on? You do not go from fully functioning healthy adult, to the complete opposite, without something being really wrong. All anyone ever wanted to do was treat the symptoms, but not try to find the cause. I had learned it did not matter what medication I took. The strength, the dose; it did not matter. They did not help.

I will admit I had a ton of help from my mom on the researching aspect. I do not know how many hours she spent online, or books rented from the library. Nights and days, she spent trying to put the puzzle together. But it was a lot. And I must thank her from the bottom of my heart for doing this, because a lot of the ideas we came up with as to what to pursue next, came from her. I believe many times she told me "What else am I supposed to do?". Meaning, how could I watch my only child suffer and not try to do all I could to help; to find answers.

One of the ideas my mom came up with was to start seeing a myofunctional therapist. I will dive deeper into precisely what this is later, with one of my therapists. But in short, its learning, retraining, and strengthening the jaw, the tongue, and different muscles in the face and mouth. Learning to chew, talk, and swallow correctly. Unbeknownst to me, the longer that my jaw was out of place, and messed up, the worse these functions got. The worse it was functioning, the more pain I was in. What did not help as well, was the amount of Botox I got into my jaw muscles trying to help with the pain, which depleted any sort of muscle mass that I had. I had a great heroin cheek look going, and not a wrinkle in sight, but sadly I did not want to become a runway model and look like I was starving for a cheeseburger.

After much research, my mom and I found out that this was a new field, and that there was not anybody in my city that dealt in depth with adults with this problem. There were therapists who dealt with children, but more for speech issues, and other issues that children sometimes have growing up. We could not find anyone that had the training to deal with an adult, and the ones that dealt with children did not want to take me on as a client. I always looked young for my age, but sadly not young enough to get an appointment.

We ended up finding a specialist who at that time was based out of Seattle, and very well known in the field.  She noticed basically every function of my jaw and face was wrong, and we started therapy. The exercises were kind of crazy looking probably for an onlooker, but I quickly realized that they were working, as I was getting better functioning, and the exercises were getting easier. I was well on my way to getting that Brad Pitt jaw line. At this point it was the summer of 2017 and my TV show of choice currently was Community, and Brooklyn Nine-Nine.

One of the suggestions that she made was getting orthodontic treatment, to help my bite, and hopefully help my jaw as well. I had been to see a few orthodontists before her recommendation, both with unsatisfying results. One would not even work with me until I was six months pain free. As I had been in serious pain for at this time almost 5 years, it was laughable that this would be possible anytime soon. I believe that he was afraid of possibly making things worse, or it was his standard protocol not to work with anyone that was in that much pain. The second person I saw, flat out told me he did not know what to do with me and did not know the course of action or treatment I should take. He was going to ask around to his fellow colleagues and try to come up with a plan. I decided against seeing him after this, as I did not want to see someone that was unsure of what to do.

Again, during my mom's research, she was able to find another orthodontist on the other side of the city, and they as well had a myofunctional therapist that worked out of the office. During our initial search, we did not find this office, so perhaps we missed it, or perhaps they had just implemented a myofunctional program.

I knew right away during the initial consultation that this was the place that I needed to go. They saw all the things wrong with my jaw and bite, but instead of being intimidated with my symptoms and what they saw, they were intrigued, and wanted to help. The first plan of action was to get invisalign, which was a relief to me as I did not want braces at 28 years of age. After having braces all of high school, I did not want to relive those memories, even though my metal smile was I am sure still captivating. Invisalign would help get my bite in proper position, and hopefully take some tension off my jaw and facial muscles. He believed that the prior splints I had, that were supposed to get my jaw back into the right place, might have contributed to my teeth and bite becoming quite bad. The difference from when I got my braces off at 18, and what it looked like now, was quite a stark contrast, it did not even look like the same person's mouth.

As well, I met with the myofunctional therapist who worked out of the office, and thankfully she was just as knowledgeable about the subject, as the therapist I was seeing online. I made the decision to see her instead as in my view it was much easier to see someone in person, and have them be able to see results and teach you exercises while right in front of you. It was also nice that she and my orthodontist would work in combination with each other. I asked her, Naurine Shah, to give a detailed description of what it is she does.

"Myofunctional therapy is described as working with the oro-facial muscles to train them for a proper function which includes rest posture, chewing, swallowing, breathing, etc. It also aims to help with oral muscle function disorders including thumb sucking, tongue thrusting, nail-biting, and mouth breathing. Many people can benefit from this type of therapy but especially if you have any kind of abnormality for lip and tongue posture as well as TMJ pain, other facial pain, and sleep issues related to breathing. Results come fast if compliance with exercises is good. Usually, you will start to see results within 2 weeks provided there are no lip or tongue ties. Typically, active treatment is for 3-6 months and then just monitoring is required periodically.

A lot of times people may think they can look up exercises on the internet, and not have to see a therapist but it's always best to contact someone who is qualified and renowned for the work that they do. Just doing random exercises does not usually help someone for a specific problem. A myofunctional therapist can make a treatment plan and have exercises that would target specific groups of muscles. It would include stretching, strengthening, and toning of the muscles. It is best to look for professional organizations that certify these individuals. IAOM is one prominent one and the certification to look for is a COM (certified Oral myologist). Only dentists, speech pathologists, and hygienists are certified at this moment. It is best to ask your orthodontist or speech-language pathologist for the referral.

In addition to myofunctional therapy, it is common for someone to get orthodontic work at the same time. Usually, orthodontics helps create space for all the muscles to achieve harmony and balance between the jaws. Chiropractors and physiotherapists are also some adjunct professionals that one may see while also getting myofunctional therapy. As this field gains more and more popularity, dentists and orthodontists are recognizing its importance. More people are getting certified and educated on the benefits of working with the muscles and not just the teeth and bones as a part of the bigger picture of oral health. More treatments are being centered around the end goal of a balanced face and function then just straight teeth."

# Chapter 8

# How Many Puzzle Pieces Are There? (2018-19)

Over the course of the next year or so, there was not all too much to write about. In the summer of 2018, the TV show of choice was Seinfeld and Curb your enthusiasm. I have seen some episodes of Seinfeld probably 50 times, but it never gets old. Before starting orthodontic treatment, I had to have 2 more tongue surgeries, I was becoming an expert! After it healed, I started with both the orthodontic treatment, and the myofunctional treatment. I could tell that things were getting much better in both departments over the course of the next year, however, I saw minimal changes in all my symptoms, which was a bit disheartening. The only thing that changed was less jaw pain, which I suppose I was happy just to have that.

It was April 2019 when the orthodontic treatment ended. My teeth were nice and straight, and my bite was ideal, and my facial muscles were functioning much better from therapy, but again, symptom wise, very minimal difference. It was at this time where I felt a lot of pressure from my parents to try and go back to work, or at least see if I could do it. I think they felt as much frustration as me with little reduction in symptoms, and in their words, they wanted me to try to get on with my life as best as I could, and for them that meant to try and work. With this treatment over with, we thought that again, we had run out of options, and maybe this was as good as I was going to get.

Of course, I knew myself, and knew what I was feeling, and had serious doubts if I could work. I had not been able to go back to my practicum at the probation office, and I had not worked part time at the grocery store since October 2015. I had started a business selling artwork, and kept quite busy with that, but I did not make near enough money to support myself.

I did make the decision to try to go back to work, and even getting to that point of just trying, was a milestone for me. I knew it was going to be very difficult, I knew it was not going to be easy, but I had to push myself to at least try. I was begging for any kind of return to normalcy in my life, and even just being able to work at my old job, would mean a lot for me. I was excited to see some of my old friends and colleagues that I had not seen in years. Some of the funniest times, jokes and stories had come from years and years of working at the grocery store with these friends. Perhaps being surrounded by produce all day brought out the best in everyone.

Unfortunately, even with my best efforts, I could only last about 5 shifts. There were so many things that were triggering worse symptoms, and my body was greatly rejecting the experience. The fluorescent lights, the continuous movement of people, the loud noises, carrying heavy loads of weight, the constant movement, all contributed to overwhelming symptoms. Many of those shifts I ended up crying in the bathroom, because of how I felt, and a lot of the tears were just out of frustration as well. Even having my friends work with me every shift and having them help me as much as I needed, was not enough.

Having to again take a leave of absence, and realize yet again, that I could not work, was a big blow mentally. It was a struggle to remain positive, to remain optimistic, and hold out hope that the future would be bright. I knew I had so much to give, so much to offer the world, but I was still marred in symptoms that left me unable to live a normal life at all. Even after all the research that my mom and I did, we were left without any answers as what we should do next. There did not seem to be a clear-cut answer, and it almost seemed like a dead end. I probably sound like a broken record, but honestly over the years it felt like there were so many dead ends. It was now the summer of 2019, and at this point I obviously still must tell you what I was watching this summer for some reason. Netflix series was the popular one, with shows like Mindhunter, The Alienist, The Sinner, and The After Life. Did I mention I watched Big Brother every summer too - But I swear the seasons get worse every year!

It was at this point that I got back in contact with a local personal trainer that had been following my story for some time. I had seen him for an initial assessment a year prior, and really wanted to start training with him as I believed he could help. Unfortunately, I could not afford to pay for the amount of sessions that I believe I needed. When he saw that I had to leave work, he reached back out to me to offer his services and told me to not worry about paying in full right off the bat.

It was a very gracious offer of him, and the next week we started training. When one thinks of personal training, a gym with heavy weights and equipment may come to mind, but this type of training was quite different. The training method is called functional patterns, and I asked my trainer, Ben Thornton to explain in depth a little bit about what it is he does, as it may seem a little complicated to the average person.

" Functional Patterns is a training system developed by Naudi Aguilar that is designed to help people walk, run, throw, stand, and breathe more effectively. By observing the movement patterns seen by elite athletes like Usain Bolt, Floyd Mayweather, Barry Sanders, Lebron James, and more, a blueprint has been developed of how high-functioning bodies move in space, and most importantly, how they can sprint efficiently and pain-free. This blueprint can be used to assess anyone's movement and guide their training/treatment in efforts to eliminate pain and improve performance.

Our bones essentially "float" in the web of tension created by all the muscles and fascia that hold the skeleton in place, and ideally that tension is well balanced from head to toe. However, in modern culture, it is extremely common for imbalances to occur all throughout the body and for people's posture, movement, and health to suffer as a result.

Functional Patterns practitioners help re-tension the body back into a balanced state by teaching client's self-massage, performing hands-on therapy, applying corrective exercises that create a stretch in one area by holding tension in another, and implementing weight training that mimics the movement patterns we use when walking, running, standing, and throwing (The "Big 4" of fundamental human movement).

FP aims to get people out of pain and discomfort by making their movements more energy-efficient, essentially improving our relationship with our most constant stressor, gravity. This can have a dramatic effect on anyone's physiological and mental health, as every single process in our body involves some sort of mechanical movement (digestion, circulation, hormone secretion, energy production, etc.). By going through FP training, many have reported a large improvement to their quality of life.

Movement is one of the primary ways we can deal with stress, but if your relationship with gravity is poor, going for a run to clear your head will only give you short-term relief and add more long-term stress to the equation. Your imbalances cause certain areas of your body to become overworked, while others become under-utilized. This reduces the range of motion you have in a joint, because the "weak" muscles can't lengthen the "tight" muscles enough.

While it's possible to improve your running speed without addressing your biomechanics, you will likely be speeding up the breakdown of your joints and ligaments due to your muscles and fascia not rebounding the impact forces of running effectively. Any FP practitioner will tell you that a marker for health and vitality is not how much you run, but how you run.

I believe that anyone can benefit from this type of training, but specifically there are a few things to look for that are common. Any muscular or joint pain is a sign that something is out of balance in the body, and the root of that imbalance likely comes from a faulty movement pattern they have had for far longer than they've had the pain. Every individual comes with a different combination of issues, and even though they might not be experiencing pain now, if they exhibit some of the common imbalances laid out below, they might be in trouble down the road, and would benefit greatly from addressing these faulty patterns.

_Anterior (Forward) Hip Shift_ – The pelvic bowl should be stacked over the ankles in standing posture to prevent pushing the centre-of-gravity forward, as that can force the spine, ribs, shoulders, and neck to compensate.

_Anterior Pelvic Tilt_ – When the pelvic bowl remains tilted forward, this compresses the lumbar spine as the low back excessively arches to keep you upright. It also represents an inability for the glutes and hamstrings to create hip extension and length in the hip flexors/quads.

_Thoracic Kyphosis/Compressed Ribs_ – Our ribs are meant to expand easily in all directions, supporting the head and shoulders and moving with our spine in fluid, elastic motion. They can only do this when the individual has balanced tension around the ribcage and a well-functioning diaphragm that can cause significant pressure in the lungs and abdomen. Many people in today's world have an inability to breathe in a manner that pulls their breastbone up and away from the front of their hips without excessively arching the lumbar spine. This results in individuals being stuck in a "slouched" position, and the implications that can have on one's health are huge.

_Forward Head Posture_ – Our skull should be nicely balanced over our shoulders, but it is common to see the head hanging in a forward position instead. This puts unnecessary strain on the back of the neck.

_Knock-knee's (Knee Valgus)_ – It is common to see one or both knee joints rotating inwards when the foot plants on the ground, especially when running and jumping. This represents poor hip connection and can lead to lots of injuries, including meniscus and ligament injuries.

_Scoliosis_ – When one's spine curves or shifts excessively to one side, it usually comes along with plenty of other imbalances such as the ones mentioned above combined with hip, ribcage, foot, and neck imbalances. It is a difficult puzzle to solve, but when you create tension and pressure in the right places, the spine can be guided back into a straighter position.

Why functional patterns over more traditional personal training and gym equipment? Unfortunately, many traditional lifting programs do not train the movement patterns you use when walking, running, and throwing. The most popular exercises are done with the feet side by side and only demand a vertical force, as opposed to the horizontal and rotational forces humans create when running. Adapting to these lifts can cause or increase imbalances, having a detrimental effect on your movement in the long-term. To better understand why, here is a quick primer on running biomechanics.

To perform a sprint, the body must cover a horizontal distance as fast as possible, meaning they will need to produce most of their force in the direction they are running (horizontally).

The body does this largely through rotation and reciprocation. To take a large step, one leg is propelled forward by the action of the opposite leg driving backwards. This reciprocating pattern is seen in the rotation of the hips, ribcage, and head as well as the swinging of the arms.

When the timing of these motions is well-coordinated, it results in roughly half of the body getting stretched by the movement of the other half. The pattern repeats itself in the opposite direction, and a stretch-recoil cycle is created that allows you to move elastically and effortlessly.

Search "Usain Bolt Slow Motion" on YouTube to see how much of a stretch he gets on his quads and hip flexors during his stride, and how the rotation of his upper body propels the motions of the legs. Human running is a beautiful display of spiraling movement when the entire body is working as one unit. If you watch a slow-motion clip of a professional baseball pitcher, or really any sport, you will notice similar patterns of movement used by high level athletes.

While many traditional exercises such as the squat, dead lift, and bench press get large activation of important sprinting muscles (like the glutes, hamstrings, and chest), the body position, patterns of activation (both legs extending at the same time), and direction of force created are completely different than how you would use those muscles when you walk or run.

Over the long-term all the vertical force traditional lifting puts on the body can result in painful compression of the hips, spine, and ribcage, which greatly hinders your ability to create horizontal force and run without pain. While FP exercises will teach you how to squat and hinge effectively while lifting heavy objects, much more emphasis is placed on the sequence of horizontal force production to walk, run, and throw efficiently. This is done using cable machines, parabolic motions with dumbbells, medicine balls, kettle bells and clubs, and precise execution of spiral movement patterns that involve the hip and ribcage rotations seen in running and throwing.

Initial exercises for the FP program often focus on static posture and the ability to create a neutral spinal alignment with proper breathing mechanics in exercises like a plank, prone cobra, or even just a standing position.

Once you have got an understanding of how to hold a strong structural integrity, two of the most foundational exercises you can perform are the stepping 1-arm row and 1-arm press. These will greatly improve the connection between your upper body and lower body, teaching the ribs to rotate in a way that helps pull the leg forward.

Many clients can feel a difference in their body after the 1st session. However, strengthening those connections, balancing the body, and learning new movement patterns is a process that takes some dedication.

The time it takes to see results is dependent on many factors; the clients pre-existing issues and their complexity, the effort outside of sessions and understanding from the client, and the experience and knowledge from the trainer.

Sometimes pain that has been present for years can be resolved in 2-4 sessions. Other times the problem is so complicated it may take 20-40 sessions to fix the issue, but the client should feel they are headed in the right direction and hopefully getting some relief throughout that period.

Many clients will invest in a 10-session package right off the bat and can make great progress in that time. Human biomechanics is a deep rabbit hole though, and if the client wants to keep improving, they can learn from a trainer for years.

There is an official map of all the Human Biomechanics Specialists in the world on www.functionalpatterns.com. There are also trainers working towards those certifications that are likely advertising their services through social media. Many may claim to offer functional training, but those who have dived deep into the Functional Patterns system will likely have the best training skill set out there.

Generally, you want practitioners that can showcase video before/after results both on themselves and their clients. Trainers can talk theory all day long and sound very convincing, but you should seek out someone who can successfully apply their knowledge on multiple bodies.

Along with functional patterns, any treatment designed to create balance in the body will be made much for effective when the dysfunctional movement patterns that created imbalances are addressed. This can include but is not limited to Chiropractic care, Cranio-sacral massage, Deep-tissue massage, Acupuncture, Dry needling, and Naturopathic medicine.

It is common for people that commit to Functional Patterns to not need those other modalities to manage their tension and pain because they feel so much better day-to-day.

In conclusion, I believe the Functional Patterns system is the future of training. It approaches the goal of optimizing the human body by taking what we know about physics, biology, chemistry, mathematics, and biomechanics, and combines them in a formulaic way that allows trainers all over the world to improve the quality of life of people that have suffered because of the dysfunction in their body's. Injured athletes, office workers, chronic pain victims, and even those with mental and physical disorders have all been benefitted from using this system.

I highly encourage anyone reading to visit the Functional Patterns Instagram and Facebook pages to see the amazing results for yourselves. On the FP website, there is a 10-week online course available that will guide you through the first steps towards moving and function pain-free, but if you are able to work 1-on-1 with a FP practitioner, that would be the best way to get started."

As you can see by his write up for me, Ben is very passionate about his work, and equally as knowledgeable. One thing that I noticed is that he was continually learning, continually advancing himself and his body in the world of functional patterns. Always trying to learn more and educate himself more on all sorts of aspects concerning the body. Because of all this, I knew that he was the right person for me to see and knew that we would get results together. *If you wish to get in contact with any of the practitioners I have mentioned, I will leave my contact information at the end of the book and pass that information along to you. *

And my intuition was right. Looking back, it was crazy to me to see just how messed up my body was. All my life I had been such an active person, playing and excelling in all sorts of sports, super flexible, and there did not seem to be a limit in terms of what I could do physically. But chronic pain had changed all this, and really took its toll on my body. Even though yes, I had bad symptoms, my body also was not moving and functioning properly either. Simple things like walking or bending over, would hurt and be very uncomfortable. I especially noticed how limited I was physically when I tried to go back to work. It was such a struggle to do any sort of movements, or lifting, and all the walking I had to do only aggravated the pain I was having. This type of dysfunction showed up right away on our initial assessment, and initial exercises. My body was totally out of wack, and not working in harmony. My head posture was very forward, my shoulders were slanted, my ribs were compressed, my lower back had a huge curve in it from a forward pelvic tilt, I had slight scoliosis, and as well like my shoulders, one hip was higher than the other.

In terms of how my body got this way, I think there were many factors.  One, being the jaw. As because my jaw was out of place for so long, it started to affect my neck muscles. Then my neck muscles started to affect my traps, and eventually it just worked its way down my body. For many years until I tore my muscles at work, I was still going to the gym and lifting weights, and as well still working in produce lifting heavy bags around all day. I think this only helped add to the dysfunctions I had. Another thing I believe happened, is that my migraines caused a forward head posture overtime. One of the things I always said was that it felt like my head weighed a thousand pounds. Thus, it was hard to keep a proper head posture, and often it would tilt a bit forward. Lastly, I believe that not being very active, and spending a lot of time sitting, laying down, sleeping, or resting, contributed as well.

I will not lie, training at first was very rough. I was constantly nauseas, constantly dry heaving and burping up stuff during the sessions, but Ben was patient with me, and I always pressed on. It felt as though I had about 8 beers before every session, and that they were not sitting quite right. Slowly but surely together we started to try to get my body back functioning properly, and hopefully, lessen some pain and symptoms along the way. I did not need a Chris Hemsworth body, I just wanted to walk and move without discomfort.

<u>Chapter 9:</u>

## Latest Findings and the Present Day (2019-20)

Other than doing this training, I was not sure what else I could do to find answers to my symptoms. While doing my artwork, and sharing my story online, I built up quite a following on Instagram, of both people that liked my art, and those that were interested in my journey. A lot of these people had chronic pain and illnesses as well. Over the years I had dozens, maybe hundreds of people message me offering advice, or things that worked for them, or even what they thought I may have, as I was still searching for answers. The chronic illness community on Instagram is truly a great community of people, and most of us have the goal is just trying to help or be there for each other as best as we can.

Over the years I had many people speculate as to what might be the root of my problems, and there were a few diseases or conditions that kept popping up. One of them was Lyme disease. After feeling like I was at yet another dead end, I started to explore more in depth about Lyme disease, and whether I fit the description. My only previous knowledge came from when Bart Simpsons teacher Edna Krabappel, had Lyme on The Simpsons.

Lyme disease is an infectious disease which is spread by ticks. The most common sign of an infection is a red rash that appears near the site of a tick bite, however not all people bitten will get this rash. Early symptoms may include fever, headache, and tiredness. If untreated symptoms may include loss of facial functioning, joint pain, severe headaches, neck stiffness, vertigo or dizziness, memory problems etc. The bacteria were first discovered in 1981, making it a relatively new infectious disease. Ticks may also carry and transmit several other parasites, or co-infections.

After much research, what I found were total descriptions of me, almost every symptom I had. But my symptoms also fit very well into a lot of other illnesses and diseases as well. I learned quickly, that just getting tested, and getting treated for Lyme, was not that easy at all. It was one of the least studied and researched diseases, and there was not even a proper diagnostic tool, it seemed to differ in every country. I learned that in Canada, the blood test to find out if you have Lyme was very flawed, and not up to date at all, about 20-30 years behind the times. There were multiple stories that I read of people getting tested in Canada, getting a negative, and then getting tested in other countries, and having it come up positive.

After asking a few friends who I knew had Lyme, what the best course of action for me to get tested was, the common consensus was getting my blood work sent to Germany. They have a world-renowned lab for tick borne diseases, and their blood tests were very thorough, having many different indicators and markers for Lyme, not just testing for one indicator like the Canada test.

The bad part about having blood work sent to Germany, was that it was not paid for under our health care system, and I could not have this done by my own doctor. I had to go to a naturopathic doctor and have everything done through her.

Even though it was costly, I made the decision to go for it, and have the testing done. Even if the test came back negative, I figured it would still be worth it, as I could cross Lyme off my list, and move onto something else to try and find answers.

After my initial appointment, my naturopathic doctor was convinced that there was a high chance I could have Lyme, just due to what my symptoms were, and the timeline of everything happening. I as well forgot that in 2012, I had a very large weird looking rash for a long time, and seemingly right after that, my symptoms slowly started. At the time, I thought the rash was from an allergy to basil, as I bought a basil plant and put the stuff on everything right around the same time the rash appeared. I was pleased as I could enjoy basil again without fearing an allergic reaction, just as I did shrimp years prior. Is my love of food starting to show?

Very soon after my initial appointment, I had my blood drawn, and sent to Germany, and would have to wait about 7-10 days for the results. I remember the day of the results very vividly. I was sitting in a waiting room, waiting to get an ultrasound. I looked down at my phone and saw that an email had come in from the lab with my results. I made a joke to myself that maybe I should not open it while in a room full of a dozen people, because maybe I would become emotional.

I opened the email. It came back positive. With multiple indicators of Lyme all coming back positive, as well as co-infections and other blood work coming back wonky as well. I could not contain the tears flowing down, and I immediately ran out of the office, and into the parking lot, where I basically collapsed against a wall. It felt like years of pent up anger, frustration, sadness, suffering all coming out at once. When you have so many symptoms, but do not know the root cause, you are constantly living on edge, constantly wondering what is wrong, and constantly questioning yourself, and everything. So many tests that I went through over the years came back normal, and just from that, I was expecting this one to come back normal as well.  Even though myself and my naturopath felt there was a high probability of a positive result, it was still very much a shock for me.

Afterwards I felt I deserved a nice lunch out, before I came home and told my parents. While chowing down, and after the initial emotions wore off, I felt a sense of calm and almost relief. And boy was I hungry.

My parents had almost the same reaction I did, and we were all very pleased that we had potentially some answers. I made the decision to get more comprehensive testing from the same lab, just to know exactly what I had, and what I would be working with moving forward. This comprehensive test came back with more Lyme markers, and I now knew that this was not just a false positive.

Normally, being diagnosed with something after years of debilitating symptoms would be an ecstatic feeling, but the more I learned about Lyme, the less I liked, and the less I felt confident I could see lessening symptoms relatively soon. Like I mentioned earlier, getting treatment for Lyme is not easy. One of the reasons for this is that, unless caught quickly, Lyme can spread throughout the body, and become harder to treat. The initial protocol is for antibiotics, but there is only a high chance of success if Lyme is caught early. At this point, it had been 7 years since my potential tick bite, and just as long having all the symptoms.

Even though I tested positive multiple times from this German test, Canada does not recognize testing from other countries, only their own. I later got tested under the Canadian test, and it came back negative. Because of this, and the lack of knowledge about Lyme by many doctors here, my positive German test results really did not matter too much in terms of getting treatment or seeing any other specialist in Canada. A lot of doctors and specialists are not aware of the faulty Lyme testing and will take other Lyme tests with a grain of salt. Anything that I wanted to do, I was basically on my own for paying for treatment.

After this positive Lyme result, I went back to my neurologist. She wanted to do a comprehensive brain MRI and was open to the idea that I could have Lyme and wanted to retest everything and compare with prior images. Sometimes Lyme will show up in imaging, sometimes it would not. She also figured since it had been 3-4 years from my last MRI, it would be good to see if anything had changed.

My MRI came back with a few abnormalities, the main one being idiopathic intracranial hypertension. Which basically means there is a build up of cerebral spinal fluid in the brain. This can be dangerous as it can cause damage to nerves in the brain, specifically the optic nerve. If the optic nerve is affected then scary visual problems can happen such as blacking out, double vision, and weird visual disturbances. It can also lead to permanent blindness. This build up of fluid can also cause severe migraines as well.

My neurologist explained that she wanted to drain and analyze this fluid. Before doing this however, we had to see if my optic nerve was being affected, so she sent me to an optomologist, a fancy term for eye specialist. He would run several tests and determine if the optic nerve was affected or not.

Happily, after testing it was determined my nerve was fine, and I was free to continue my journey to become a fighter pilot. I went back to the neurologist expecting to book an appointment to drain the fluid build up. Weirdly though, her opinion had changed, and I am unsure if it was because of the optimologist report, or just a change of heart. Because now she did not want to drain this fluid. I tried to ask why and get some answers, but her responses weren't that clear to me, and she basically said unless I wanted to try different meds that there wasn't anything else she could do for me at this time. There was a new migraine drug on the market I wanted to try, but she claimed that it would interact with my current medication, so I could not try it.

Something did not seem right with me, so I did some research on my own about the subject. Everywhere I looked, on all reputable websites, it clearly stated that leaving this fluid is not something that should be done, especially if a patient has severe symptoms, which I did. It as well stated that regular checkups should happen, where the eyes, nerves, and symptoms were regularly checked for any change. She did not mention any of that either.

I decided to get a second opinion from another neurologist who confirmed everything that I thought. He said the fluid should not be left, and in the very least, should be analyzed and tested as well. He then booked me an appointment for this procedure. He also mentioned that the drug I had wanted to try, with his knowledge, did not interact with my medication. In fact, it barely interacted with any other drugs at all.

It was a little concerning that two neurologists would have such differing opinions on what to do given certain findings, and about drugs. But from my years of experience with the medical system at this point, it did not surprise me. I obviously had learned to take matters into my own hands, do my own research, and get other opinions before deciding what path to take. I was just happy that things would hopefully be moving forward, not stagnant, or backward.

Believe it or not, this brings us to the present day. Due to the worldwide pandemic, my Lyme treatment has been pushed off. The plan was to initially try out a bunch of antibiotics and see if I had any noticeable results. But based off my knowledge, and from other Lyme friends' experiences, I am not expecting it to work, but it is worth a try. After this, there is no protocol for what the treatment for Lyme should be. There are a number of different treatments, but most of the effective ones seem to be out of country, and obviously not covered, and quite pricey. If I must go this route, I will. I will do anything that I can to try and feel better. Again, there are lots of treatments, pills, and therapies that claim to help with symptoms of Lyme, but I want to get rid of it, or put it into remission. There is a clinic in, again Germany (Those damn smart Germans), that has a high rate of successfully getting rid of Lyme. I had a friend I met online with Lyme, recently go there for treatment with great results, seemingly putting it into remission, so it is always a potential option for the future.

There of course is the hope that draining the build up of fluid in my brain will provide some migraine relief, or at the very least, provide us with a bit more information of what is going on. As well I have hopes that this new migraine medication will be effective. For some people I know, it has been life changing, with relatively no side effects, so my fingers are crossed. However, this drug is very new, and still very pricey. Just the normal cost of business for someone with a chronic condition!

Where my symptoms came from, and what caused certain things, I do not think I will ever know. Did the jaw fracture cause any issues? How did I get vestibular nerve damage? How much of my symptoms are from my jaw being messed up? How did my jaw become that bad in the first place? How many of my symptoms are from Lyme disease? How many of them are from fluid build up in my head? Did the many concussions I had as a child contribute to anything? Honestly, I think everything contributed to a perfect storm sort of situation, and it is probably why my situation is so complex, and hard to treat.

In terms of how I feel today, everyday is different, and it vastly depends on the symptoms I am having that day. If they are severe, I am very limited, not able to do much at all other than just trying to make it through the day. If symptoms are reduced, it is almost as if I am back to normal. I can go out with friends, I am able to engage in conversations, I have an appetite, and am able to think clearly. I can do whatever I like, without any boundaries. These really good days are rare, maybe only a couple a month, but they feel almost angelic and magical, and give me hope that one day I can have that feeling all the time. Most of the time my symptoms are in between severe and good.

I am continuing to train with Ben, and over the past year, we have seen great results, and my body is functioning way better than it has throughout my journey. It is the single best thing I have done for myself. I can walk long distances without much pain, and overall things are moving better, however there is still much work to go. I am forever grateful for him reaching out to me and using me as sort of a learning tool for himself. I am excited for every session, and even more excited about what progress we can make in the future. I still miss training the old fashion way at the gym, and my bigger muscles from yester year, but there's more important things in life. I am also still continually seeing the other therapists and practitioners mentioned, as they have been the only ones, I have seen that have helped my symptoms.

I still deal with vertigo, chronic pain, intense migraines, and dizziness, and nausea every single day. Along with these symptoms comes intense brain fog where it can be hard to think and speak coherently at times. My body is still in a state of fight or flight. Everything feels racy, sort of like you have had a huge shot of caffeine all day long. It can make it hard just to catch your breath. Lately I have noticed a lot more joint pain, along with my joints popping and cracking and sometimes dislocating. There have been many times where my knee or shoulder will pop out, and I will have to pop it back in. I am still waiting for my permanent gig to join the circus!

My day to day life is not that exciting. When I wake up, usually my symptoms are at their worst, so I spend this time relaxing, meditating, doing breathing exercises, stretching, self massage on certain muscles, anything to calm my system and get ready for the day. I will usually take out my dog, Finn, for a walk or two, go to any appointments I may have, and then do some work for my business. Answer emails, messages, comments, and then get down to some artwork. Thankfully, business has remained constant over the years. At night usually I will watch sports, spend time with friends or talk over the phone, or play video games. Usually late at night is when I have been writing this book. For some reason that is when I can think more clearly, and I have written more words past midnight than any other time. Of course, if symptoms are bad you can replace everything I just wrote in this paragraph, and instead i'll have many ice packs going, trying to remain in complete darkness and silence. I prefer the first part! There are days that I have that are still very bad, and can be super overwhelming, both mentally and physically. But how do I get through these days? What have I learned on my journey about how to cope with chronic pain and illness? Well you are in luck, since that is what part two of the book is about!

## Chapter 10: Noting

Now that you have read the entirety of my journey, you might ask yourself "how does one continue on with life while going through all of that?". Sometimes I ask myself the same question. If I really think back and realize what I have been through, it amazes me that I am still here. Perhaps a new marvel comic book hero is in the works. I need a good comic book name, maybe Pain Train? Lyme Tyme? Hmmm, I need to think of something better.

Since this journey of mine has lasted so long, and the symptoms have always been here in some degree or another every day, I have had to learn and adapt along the way. This part of the book explains what I have learned and strategies that I have incorporated into my life to make living more manageable. I think it is important to say that these are strategies that worked for me, and they may not work for everybody. But I also think it is important to say that I believe these strategies are not just to get through chronic pain. They can be useful for almost anybody who is going through anything, or if you just want to live a better life and become the best version of you.

When my journey started, I was told by everybody, and believed myself, that my symptoms would just be a temporary thing. My doctors said it could be something that will eventually pass, and my parents tried to assure me by saying one day I may wake up and it would be gone. For a long time, almost the first couple years, I believed that any day it would be over, and I would go back to my normal life. I was not prepared at all to deal with the idea that the pain and symptoms I was dealing with would be chronic, and something I could potentially be dealing with for a long time.

And that is the biggest difficulty that I have dealt with throughout my journey, the chronic part. My day always starts out with a bang. I wake up, and my pain and symptoms hit me like a brick. Radiating and stabbing pain all over my face, jaw, and head. Nausea, dizziness, and a racing heart. It literally takes my breath away, much like a good tiramisu. It takes a few minutes to just even grasp the situation, like an algebra equation. I have dealt with this for years waking up feeling this way. Dealing with it for one day would be bad, but after hundreds and now into the thousands, it takes its' toll not only physically, but mentally -  and the mental side is where we are going to start down the long and winding road of things that I have learned.

Explaining what chronic pain feels like to someone who has not experienced it, is hard. Most of us at some point in our lives will experience some sort of physical pain. But it is usually for a short duration. We usually know the cause; we know how to fix it and when it should subside, and if needed, drugs usually work well until the severe part is over. But of course, with chronic pain, it is never over - that day may never come. It is like new seasons of Grey's Anatomy; it just keeps going and going. After a certain number of days and amount of time, chronic pain starts to affect you mentally. Chronic pain eventually breaks you. It starts to take over you; take over all your thoughts.  It makes you scared; it wants you to fear it. It is so easy to go down a dark path of thoughts. "Why do I have to suffer?", "What did I do to deserve this?", "What is the point of all this?", "Will I ever get better?", "I don't know if I can take this any longer", "Why me?", and during the darkest of times, "I don't want to live anymore. I don't want to go through this anymore, I hate my life". These are such natural thoughts to have while dealing with chronic issues. These are thoughts I had almost every day. But I learned overtime, that the more you think about the pain, the despair, and the anger, the more you resist and fight the pain, the stronger it becomes. It is like the Blob, that eats up everything in its' path, and just gets bigger and stronger.  Soon the Blob eats the whole town, and you are like, damn this Blob is powerful!

It is hard and believe me I still struggle with the idea of this, but to fight the Blob, you must accept the Blob. Make the Blob part of your life. Embrace it. The Blob is ugly, oh man is it ever. You hate the Blob, but if you make friends with it, it is easier for you to tolerate it. OK, we remember that the Blob is chronic pain, right? Anyways, we must change our relationship with pain, and stop fighting it.

But how do we do this? The Blob is ever powerful. The first step is changing our thought patterns. If we buy into the fact that we cannot do anything, that our life is ruined, that we do not want to live anymore, over time you start to believe those things. Your mind and body give in. It's like the old saying my Mom, the great philosopher, used to say, "If you look in the mirror every day and tell yourself you are ugly, you become ugly". You must have the self-awareness to realize that these thoughts are only hurting you, even if you completely agree with them.

What I did not realize, was that I was thinking of pain 24/7. It was on my mind all the time. Whatever I did or thought about, it was there, of course naturally, in a negative way. I forgot what it was like to have normal thoughts, to go on with your day taking things one step at a time. A minute excerpt of my thoughts could include, "Oh let's check out the sports section and look up some baseball scores. Ugh trying to read this is making me dizzy. I cannot believe I can barely read this. Ok I have to let the dog outside. Oh, wow the sunlight is so bright, it is hurting my eyes. I want to go out and play with him in the yard, but I better close the door, the sun is making my migraine worse. Why can't I even enjoy some sunlight? I miss the days of sitting on the beach in Mexico soaking up the sun, but instead I am suffering and cannot even leave the house. My head's so bad I better lay down." As you can see, even simple tasks that I was doing, pain would dominate the dialogue in my head, I had a negative relationship with it, and I was letting it win.

A simple technique I learned is the idea of noting. Thankfully, this is not like taking notes in English class. What we must realize is that it is perfectly normal for thoughts about pain to arise. We cannot help the fact that this is going to happen. But we can help how we interact with these thoughts. Instead of buying into them, and going down a dark path, we can simply choose to acknowledge the thought, note it, and move on.

For example, say I am letting the dog out. But when the sunlight hits and I start feeling pain and thinking about it, instead of going down the path of thoughts like I did in the example above, we change our course of thinking. We say to ourselves, "Ok am I thinking about the pain, or feeling the pain? I am both thinking and feeling it. "And there it is noted. And after that we move on without diving into it more. We go onto the next train of thought which could be, "I should grab a refreshing Dr. Pepper, with 23 unique flavours in one can. Maybe a sandwich too. How old is this meat?"

So that is the concept, and really, it is as simple as that. We do not need to make it any more complicated. Whenever we think of pain, or anything that relates to it, we simply say to ourselves "Thinking" and then move onto another thought.

Similarly, whenever we feel pain, or symptoms or sensations in our body relating to it, we say to ourselves "Feeling" and then move onto another thought.

It takes time, and practice, but this noting technique will steer your mind clear of thinking about pain too in-depth. Steer your mind clear of catastrophic thinking, which increases your resistance to what you are feeling or thinking. It is amazing at the start to realize just how much you are thinking about it all day, and your day will be filled with noting these thoughts or feelings. But, overtime, your mind will change its' behaviour, and you will notice you start thinking about it less and less, and thus note less and less.

Chronic pain tells you all sorts of crazy wives tales, things that aren't true but that he wants you to believe, like the Uncle who drinks too much booze and tells conspiracy theories (Not a reference to you Uncle Ken, drink up!) But instead of cozying up to your Uncle to hear more, you need to change your relationship with him. You cannot get rid of him, but you can make the step to stop listening to him too in-depth.

Over time you will start to notice a change. You will notice the pain and the symptoms, but you will not buy into them. You will not for the next 30 minutes think of how shitty things are. You will be able to say alright yeah, I feel the pain, but that is okay.  And move on. Learning to accept the pain, the Blob, not fight it, not dive into thinking about it, in turn will decrease the blobs power.

<u>Chapter 11:</u>

## Mindfulness

You may ask yourself, "But Ryan, how does someone transition from thinking of their pain all day, to thinking of normal thoughts such as why do people eat at Taco Bell and how is Dwayne the Rock Johnson in literally every movie?" Again, it is a simple concept, but one that will take time to become a natural everyday part of your life. This is the concept of mindfulness.

Now for some people, when they hear this word, it may garner thoughts of a monk meditating beside a llama on the hillside. Yes, that does sound peaceful, but mindfulness can be achieved by anyone. Now remember the previous chapter, where I listed common thoughts, I had on a day to day basis while dealing with chronic pain? It is also common for one to have thoughts that do not pertain to the present moment. These can include, "Remember how great my life was without pain? Everything was so easy, and I miss those times so much. I miss the person I used to be I miss how life used to be." As we can see, these thoughts are all about the past.

It is so easy to fantasize when the present moment seems so hard, and so terrible. Your mind almost automatically goes and thinks about better times. However, it is so natural to romanticize the past, and make it seem better than it was. Was the past better when I was not living with chronic pain? Of course, but I was still dealing with a lot of other things, problems, and issues that life threw at me.  There are hardly any prolonged moments in life where we are not going through rough moments, and hard times. Thinking about the past and wishing to be the person you used to be or romanticizing about the memories is only making the present moment even harder to deal with. While thinking of positive memories is good, wishing to go back to the way things were, is bad. We must remember that you cannot change the past, you cannot go back. Life moves on, and we must as well.

On the other hand, we may have thoughts about the future too. These can include, "I can't picture my life in the future still living like this. How am I going to survive? My life is going to be so terrible if I have to live the rest of my life like this. How will I make it to my appointment on Friday? Will I ever meet a significant other being like this? Will I ever have kids? Will my life ever be normal?"  As you can see, obviously these thoughts are very negative, and very hyperbolic and catastrophic. But these thoughts and questions are also impossible to know the answer to in the present moment. The future is so uncertain, you do not know what is going to happen, and you cannot predict it. Thinking about the future in this way only brings upon stress and anxiety.

This brings us back to the concept of mindfulness. In short, it is living in the present moment. Not thinking about the past, or the future, but living in the now. For me, all the thoughts listed in the previous paragraphs were very common. I was not living in the present moment, I was stuck in the past, and always thinking about the future in a negative light. I had to learn to stop this way of thinking and learn to live in the present again. It is impossible not to think about the future or the past, and I am not saying to never do that, but we must change our relationship with these senses of time, think about them in a positive light, but make sure we are mostly in the present.

One of the simple tricks to mindfulness is to use all your senses at a given time, to ground yourself, and to bring yourself to the present moment. What do I smell? What sounds am I hearing? What am I touching and how does it feel? What do I taste and what am I looking at? Answering these questions may take some time, but that is a good thing. We want to analyze our senses; we want to explore these sensations that we are having. Unfortunately, while doing this you may realize, man I stink I need a shower, or, how long has this spinach been in my teeth? In any given moment in our lives our senses are bombarded. We can often hear sounds from everywhere, tons of things around us that we can touch and smell and look at. If we spend our time thinking about these things, there is no time, or room to be thinking about anything else.

It seems more and more these days that people are not living in the present moment. They are not appreciating the little things that make up a day. We always seem to be rushing from one place or another, always thinking of the next thing we must do. Instead of sitting and enjoying a moment of peace, we spend that time on our phones. When we have a conversation with someone, we are not engaged, and our minds are elsewhere, sometimes not even listening to what the other person is saying. Mindfulness over time starts to change all these things.

# Chapter 12:

## Leaning on Prior Experiences

Both strategies play a significant role in keeping yourself in a positive, optimistic outlook. Having an optimistic view of yourself, your prognosis, and the world, despite what may be going on, and the challenges you may face, is so important in the mental side of chronic pain.

What can also help you to remain positive, and to let you know that you can make it through the roughest of times, is drawing on prior experiences, and the knowledge and wisdom you may have gained through other difficult moments in your life. So many people have asked how I remain so upbeat while dealing with so much. As mentioned earlier, most of the time if you saw me, I would be cracking jokes, laughing, smiling, and no one would have any idea of the things that I go through. My little secret!

While thinking of why I was this way, I reflected on prior events in my life, challenges that I faced. When I was about 11 years old, I suffered 3 concussions in a span of a year, which left me with terrible post-concussion symptoms, where I missed almost all of grade 5. It is hard to remember much of this time as it seems all hazy. I do remember always feeling sick to my stomach, always having issues with zoning out and being tired. I dealt with headaches and dizziness and had personality changes as well. I suddenly became OCD about certain things, such as obsessive hand washing, not touching door handles, being deathly afraid of going to any sort of doctor or dentist. I was paranoid about a lot of things. This was a stark contrast to how I was before the concussions, and these symptoms lasted awhile. There was not much knowledge about concussions back then and of course these behaviours and symptoms were written off as just a phase, or things that would go away.

Because of the symptoms I was experiencing, I dealt with severe bullying, so bad that I was on the verge of transferring schools a few times. Many days I would come home crying, but there was not much anyone could do to help the situation. Previous best friends that I had, no longer wanted to hang out with me, and there was a period where I felt all alone. I remember walking the halls at lunch time during junior high, looking for anyone that would want to hang out with me.

Sadly, it seemed, everyone had their cliques, and because of the bullying, I did not have the confidence to start new friendships, as I was afraid of being hurt more than I already was. I spent a lot of lunches by myself, sometimes I would walk around the community around the school to pass the time, or save up a few dollars to buy a bagel at Tim Horton's - sesame seed bagel, toasted, with butter — so nutritious!. In the wintertime, I would just buy a coffee to keep my hands warm for the walk back. The employees thought I was so grownup and mature getting a coffee, but I would never drink it as I hated the taste. I sure fooled them!

As time passed, the confidence I had in myself, only shrunk. I had a hard time even keeping eye contact with people and would look at the ground. I was convinced that nobody wanted to be my friend, and that I was different and weird. I was convinced that any problems that my friends or family had, were because of me. I blamed myself for everything. My only goal was to survive that given day and move onto the next one.

You may ask how these experiences would affect how I deal with my chronic pain and symptoms today. Those were challenges that I had to go through at a young age, and overcome, and made me a stronger person. They let me know that I could get through anything. It also laid the groundwork and helped me understand the most personal growth that we as humans achieve, is unfortunately usually when we are faced with hard times and suffering. As hard as those junior high times were, things did get better, and I learned so much. But they only got better when I started to actively seek out ways to improve my life; it got better when I changed my outlook on myself and on the world. It took many years to overcome the confidence issues I had, and many more to learn to love myself and who I am. But things did get better; I got through those tough times and grew as a person.

So now, instead of focusing on all of the bad things that have happened, I remember that I have gotten through tough times before, and I think of all the things that I have learned through this medical journey. It has made me a better person, a better friend, a better son. I have gained insight and perspective that I would have never gained otherwise. It has taught me about what is important in life, and helped in gaining even more confidence and being happy with who I am. It has made me stronger than I ever thought I could ever be. Most importantly,

I expanded my bagel horizon, and now get an everything bagel toasted with cream cheese.

If I remember all those things and remind myself, it makes each day easier to get through. As I mentioned before, it is so easy to get down on life, and yourself when dealing with chronic pain. But if I think in-depth about all the struggles, all the things I have missed out on, and the uncertainty of the future, I will never be happy, and I will never be upbeat. I must try to make the most out of this situation I am in, and learn all that I can, and keep thinking of all the positives that have come from this situation. There is going to be hard days, days where no matter how hard I try I cannot help but be overwhelmed and sad. But I have had days where the pain has been reduced, where everything I've been through seems worth it - that is the feeling that I think about, strive, and work towards achieving every day.

# Chapter 13:

## Distraction

What is this? More tricks on how to deal with chronic pain? Yes, they call me the David Copperfield of pain. But this concept is more of an obvious one, than a trick, and that is the art of distraction and keeping busy.

Previously I had talked about all the bad thoughts that can happen while dealing with chronic pain, and I realized that these thoughts came only at certain times, and that is when I wasn't busy, or my mind wasn't occupied. When this happens, my mind was free to wander, and as I described earlier, it wandered into some dark caves; spacious, wet, and murky caves. Bats, I think there were lots of bats too.

Due to my symptoms, I was robbed of everything that I used to like to do. Playing sports, being active, working out, going out to bars and clubs, and progressing in post-secondary education, these were things that I could not do anymore and these were things that occupied pretty much my whole life before. I was at a loss initially of how I could spend my time, everything seemed so hard, strenuous, and difficult. Everything also seemed so boring. But I had to reinvent myself, I had to learn what I was capable of, and activities and hobbies that I could do even if I were feeling bad.

First off, I wanted to make sure the activities that I was doing, would also help me both physically and mentally. I didn't just want to waste time, I wanted to learn, I wanted to do things that would make me feel better, I wanted to do things that would help me grow as a person. Some of the hobbies I got into included yoga, meditation, reading, writing, art, learning Spanish, and walking all sorts of trails all over my city. I also wanted to keep my mind sharp and stimulated so I spent time doing crossword puzzles, Sudoku, playing Trivial Pursuit, and other board and video games that used knowledge or strategy. While doing all these activities, my mind was busy, and I was distracted from the pain, and all the emotions that come with it. I was too busy to jump down into the deep dark caves of the mind.

This is how I started my journey with art. It was Mother's Day 2017, and I wanted to do something homemade and special for all the mothers in my family. I was cleaning my room and found an old watercolour set that must have belonged to a much younger, innocent, spikey haired me. Seriously, what was with the amount of rock-hard hair gel used in 2006? I could have poked someone's eye out. Anyways, I had always liked to paint, create things, and loved doing art in middle school, but I never really had the patience or time to learn more in-depth. I thought this could be something that could distract me and keep me busy for a bit. I sat down, and even through all the pain and vertigo, was able to create a resemblance of some flowers, mountains, and rivers. I am not very active on social media, so I am not sure what gave me the urge to post these not so great pieces, but I did, and I was flooded with requests from friends to do paintings for them as well.

What started off that innocently, and small, turned into a full-fledged small business for me within months, and where to date I have done hundreds of pieces, all different mediums, all difference sizes, and of all different subjects. When I started to get orders, I wanted to get better, I wanted to learn more. So, I practiced, I looked up lessons on YouTube, I picked up and bought all sorts of different materials and found what worked for me. Thanks to Instagram I was able to connect with a wider audience and started shipping pieces around the world. Because I was unable to work a normal job, art provided me with an income and something to help pay off some of my medical expenses.

At the very same time I started this business, I wrote a blog story about the medical journey that I was on. Writing had always been something that I enjoyed doing and excelled anytime we had essays or writing projects in school. At the time I felt the urge, and the need, to write out all that I had been through, in a way hoping that it would be therapeutic. At first, it was only intended for me, something of an exercise to ease my mind -- to perhaps relive, and realize all the things I had went through, and to keep pushing on. After crying my eyes out writing the story (part of which is in this book), it felt like a huge weight had been lifted off my shoulders. After showing a few friends and family members, they encouraged me to share my story on my social media pages.

Because of the exposure my Instagram account was getting from the art, my blog post was read by tens of thousands of people, and I have received messages from all over the world thanking me for sharing my story, wishing me well, and in a lot of cases, people sharing their own medical story with me. It was a bit of a whirlwind but not too long after, my art and medical story was featured in both the local newspaper, and the local television news.  I have got to say, seeing yourself on TV is more embarrassing than I expected, has my voice always been this nasally? Haha.

I felt the need to continue to write about my experiences, and started doing small 500-word posts on Instagram about my journey, things I have learned, things I have been through, etc. Again, each post seemed to connect with a lot of people, and that is where the idea to put everything together in a book came from. So, a big thank you to my 20k-ish followers for continuing to motivate and push me.

Wooooosh, what a journey. And it all started because I just wanted to keep myself busy for a few days doing a few paintings for Mother's Day. Look what it turned into; that is the crazy thing about starting new hobbies or diving into existing hobbies more seriously. You never know what can happen. You never know how far you can take it. Both art and writing have taken up so much of my time, but it feels like time well spent, that it has been worth all the hours and days I have put in.

But I digress from my own journey. Back to the main point of this chapter, which was the art of distraction, and keeping yourself busy. It is so easy to be complacent and give into being a procrastinator. And I should know. All my life all I ever heard from teachers was, "Could be an exceptional student if he applied himself." But when we lounge around, not doing much of anything, for prolonged periods, it is not good for our mental health, especially if we are dealing with pain, or any other illness. It seems as we get older, we have less and less time for hobbies and activities, but I encourage you to find that time; it is more important than you might realize. You may find something that you like, even love. You may find something that brings you happiness, peace, joy, and gives you something to look forward to. A passion. You may also connect with others that share this same type of passion and make new friends and connections. Do not limit yourself; do things you love but also try out new things, expand your mind, keep learning, and keep exploring.

# Chapter 14:

## Unhealthy Distractions

Now you may realize that when I talked about distractions and keeping busy, I talked about hobbies, or activities that are physically or mentally stimulating. That is because they have positive effects and are beneficial to one who is suffering. But there are also things that are distracting but have negative consequences or effects.

The big one is of course social media and being on your phone. I do not need to go into a big rant about how bad social media and excessive phone use can be, because by now, most of us are aware of how it can impact your mental health. But, when you add dealing with chronic pain or illness into the equation, it can make it much more harmful. On social media, all you are seeing are the things people want you to see, the best sides of them, the best pictures of them, the most exciting things that they are doing, etc. This gives off the impression of how much fun they are having, how many exciting things that they are doing, and how beautiful they are. But as we know, photos can be filtered and doctored, and no one's life is a constant good time and party, even the Kardashians. But, being bombarded with these images, when you are so limited in what you can do, can be demoralizing. Initially, that is what happened with me. I saw pictures of all my friends having fun, on holidays, travelling, getting married, having babies (some looking like Danny DeVito!), and all their nights out having fun.

Here I was just struggling to make it through a given day where I was not able to do any of those things, and I was not sure when I would be able to. Because of how much free time I had, it was so easy to distract myself with checking up on social media. It took no effort, I could lie on the couch, it wasn't straining in anyway, and all I had to do was unlock my phone and I could keep busy for as long as I wanted. But in the end, it left me feeling much worse about the situation I was in. I had to focus on myself, on the small little achievements that I was able to do, and not on everyone else. My life was so much different than everyone else's. Nobody I knew was dealing with what I was dealing with, so comparing me to everyone else was being very unfair.

I will also group television in this same paragraph, as it fits a similar mould as social media. It offers nothing stimulating and beneficial unless you are watching documentaries and learning. Of course, I am not saying to remove TV, social media, or phone use completely from your life, but to use in moderation. The way I learned to control my usage was installing an app on my phone that kept track of how long I was on my phone that day, and how many times I unlocked it. Initially I got a baseline of how much time I was on it, and then gradually reduced this number overtime, and setting a new goal over and over again. It may take time to get used to using your phone less, as for many it is somewhat of an addiction. But when you do, you will notice the benefits.

The other thing I learned to do was, make sure that whoever I was following on social media was not being a detriment to my mental health.  Over the years social media has shifted to less about connecting with your friends and more about celebrities, famous athletes, and people, and as well as influencers. However, we know nothing about these people, and much of what they post are doctored pictures of themselves, photo shopped, or real-life photo shopped with lip fillers, Botox etc. Guys using steroids and lots of drugs to get that jacked but lean look. They try to sell us dumb products, and of course usually sharing only their happiest moments. But what are we admiring about celebrities? Their looks, lifestyle, and seemingly their happiness?  Why are we following them? Just so we are the first to hear the latest news and gossip and see their latest picture?  We only know what they want us to see and know, and everything they post is calculated. Most everything is driven by money.

In turn, we are almost geared to feel bad about ourselves, because we do not have what they do. We end up ourselves trying to be like them. Not enjoying food because we feel we always must be on a diet, not enjoying working out because we have not hit our goal weight, or we are not jacked enough yet. Obsessing about taking pictures and videos, but not for ourselves, but for our followers, thinking one day maybe we will be Instagram famous too. People spend more time trying to seem like they have a great life, than putting in the effort to achieve one. Both genders seem to feel the need to post selfies and half nude pictures, almost for self-validation. We learn to only post and share the best happiest moments, but life has all sorts of moments, good, bad, and ugly.

Social media has all sorts of great things about it, but we just need to be aware of who we are following, how much time we are spending on it, and how it makes us feel. For me, I wanted to follow people like me, who had chronic issues, and shared their struggles, triumphs, and journey. This made me feel so much less alone, and I really connected with a lot of people, and made a lot of friends. There are some great Instagram accounts, and one that I am an ambassador for is thechronicloveclub. This account shares small stories of people who are going through all kinds of chronic issues. In their own words they describe what they go through, their struggles, but as well their accomplishments, and what they have learned. It is amazing to read these stories every day, and see the resiliency that these people have, and it pushes and motivates me. The good side of social media is that these people's voices would be so rarely heard otherwise. In our day to day life, we rarely run into people with chronic health issues, and even if we do run into them, it is often hard to know the extent to what they are going through. I love following pages like this because it breaks the stigma of staying silent about our struggles and gives a voice to a sometimes forgotten about group.

# Chapter 15:

## Relationships

You might notice that I did not mention relationships with friends or family as ways to distract yourself or keep busy, and this is on purpose. In some situations, they can be the best way to deal with everything, and in some situations, it can also make things worse.

Before I dive into this dynamic, I want to be clear that what I think is very important is that people learn how to deal with their chronic pain/illness, on their own. Nobody knows what or how you are feeling better than you do. It is so easy to rely on others to make yourself feel better, whether you are in pain or not. But, in order to get the most out of your relationships with others, and in order to deal with your relationship with chronic pain better, it is helpful to be able to deal with the hard times without the help of anyone else. To give you an analogy, I will use the example of smoking. Say that you are out of cigarettes, and you are really craving one. You do not know how you are going to make it through the next little while without one. You know that if you call up someone, a friend or family member, they will have a cigarette for you, and you will get your fix. You never have to deal with going a long time without one and learning the coping mechanisms to get through that feeling of really craving one. Your friends and family act as enablers, always providing that cigarette, but in reality, they are keeping you addicted, keeping you craving that next cigarette.

Now some of you may be like, Ryan, you have lost your mind with this analogy but hear me out. Running immediately to your friends and family when you are having a rough time, and having them comfort you, is the cigarette. If they keep providing you with that comfort, that cigarette, the more times you will run to them when any urge hits. But running to them, prevents you from learning any coping mechanisms of your own to deal with what is going on, keeping you "addicted".

As you will see in upcoming chapters, having chronic pain impacts those around you so much. They are living through it with you. But it can be just as hard on them as it is on you. Watching someone suffer is not easy, especially if it is chronic. Taking care of someone is again, not easy, especially if chronic. If your entirety of your relationship with a family member or friend is having them be a comfort to you, or having them take care of you, it can be a real strain on the relationship. Both parties can end up feeling all sorts of emotions which can be taken out on each other. The relationship can become toxic.

This brings me back to the point of learning how to deal with the pain without someone there for you. When someone else comforts us, it hinders our ability to learn how to deal with it on our own. Hinders our ability to learn coping skills, learn self-awareness, and learn how to be independent. When we can do this, our relationships with others will be healthier, and the relationship will not be all about pain. This leads to much more normal relationships which will benefit the mental health for everyone involved.

In my own experience I never relied on others to comfort me, and always tried to keep what I was going through out of all my relationships. But I could see that when times were rough, it affected all those that were close to me. In the beginning, I did not have the tools to mentally deal with what I was going through, but overtime, learned on my own what worked for me and what did not. I still to this day have so many hard days, and so many times where I could make that the focal point of my conversations with others. So many times, where I could run and cry to someone and be comforted. Sometimes I do, but I have the self-awareness to know that this will not help anyone if I make it a common occurrence.

If I start to feel overwhelmed, instead of running to my dad, I must think, okay let us try to deal with this on my own, and let's meditate. After that, let's go for a walk and be outside in nature. After that, okay maybe let us distract myself by doing some art. After doing this I may feel better and then maybe I will be able to play a game of cards with my dad but have that quality time with him without him watching me in distress. Instead of him comforting me, we can play and talk about what dumb meme we saw on the internet today and have a laugh.

Friends and family play a vital role in anyone's life if they are dealing with something. But it is only beneficial if the relationship remains healthy. If it is a toxic environment, it can sometimes make things worse.

After writing this last part, and posting it, I received a bit of backlash on instagram, from others who did not see eye to eye with me on what I was trying to say. And that is okay. Its healthy to have a dialogue with each other and try to learn or try to understand better what a person is trying to say. I am definitely not saying to never ask for help from others. I am not saying to hide or feel bad if you have issues where you feel you need someone. I unfortunately know all too well the feeling of not being believed, wanting to hide how I really feel, not wanting to ask for help because I did not want to bother people. I know the feeling of being left out, feeling all alone, and feeling like I have no one who understands me, or gets me. I know just how badly someone having there for me on a bad day made all the difference in the world.

The point I am trying to make is that sometimes a vicious cycle can happen where we are relying on other people too much to make us feel better, and in turn this is actually making us feel worse and even more dependent. Obviously, every person is different, and everybody who has chronic issues has needs that are different. Sometimes we have no choice but to ask for help and that is okay, there is nothing wrong with that.

My experience with friendships while dealing with chronic pain is a bit of a mixed bag. When all these symptoms started for me, I was 22-23 years old, almost done university, was not dating, and had many friends that I had met through all different periods of my life. I quickly learned that with what I was dealing with, having a normal friendship was impossible. I was so limited in what I could do, where I could go. Planning something was difficult as symptoms varied so much day to day. As I mentioned earlier, I was almost afraid of people seeing me in the condition that I was in.

It did not help that I heard all the gossip about me. "I think he's just exaggerating what he's going through or making some of it up" "He should just man up, it can't be that bad, he looks fine to me".

I felt like I was being judged by a lot of people, or not taken seriously, and there were quite a few friends who had no empathy or did not seem to care. Friends that never even asked how I was doing and some friends that I have not even heard from since this whole thing started for me. I guess that would declassify them as friends after this long.

Of course, initially this hurt me, as I always tried to be the best friend I could to others, and it was feeling like I was not getting the same treatment in return. Even when others knew how bad I was feeling, I was still only asked to go out and drink and party, but not asked to do anything else. As if that was the extent of the friendship. But I had to remember that I was still so young, and that is what a lot of friendships revolved around. I also learned overtime that it was easier for people to back away and distance themselves from me, because they did not know what to do or say, or how to act. It is not easy being friends with someone with chronic pain. At the end of the day, I had to again remember that I needed to be focusing on myself and my road to recovery, and not analyzing friendships. I could not force people to come on this journey with me.

There have been many people along the way that I have met and became friends with, but only because we shared one common thing, which was chronic pain or illness. Initially I was so relieved to have close friends who knew somewhat what I was dealing with. But, overtime, some of these friendships I could see were toxic to my own healing. Dealing with others problems, both mental and physical, on top of my own, sometimes proved to be too much for me to handle, especially when those people made it a very common occurrence to run to me when things were bad. I learned strategies to deal with what I was going through, but, in the relationships that were toxic, those friends did not know how to deal, and could not see how they were behaving was bringing everyone down with them. It was hard, but I had to let some of those friends go when I realized that the relationship would never be normal.

Thankfully, I always had a few close friends to turn to if I needed them for any reason. To talk, to distract me, to make me feel better. I always tried to be conscious and always make the friendship equally about them as it was about me. In the end, having chronic pain made some of my friendships and bonds even closer.

<u>Chapter 16:</u>

## Goal Setting

As I wrote earlier, for much of my life, I was a procrastinator. I always took the easy road. Now the old king of procrastination still has not left his throne completely, but I am slowly working towards becoming better at this. It is difficult to change a lifetime of bad habits overnight, but you can start slowly. One of the things that I found helpful in terms of procrastinating less, and doing more, is making short term and long term goals, writing these down, and going through them, revising them, and checking them off constantly. When you are dealing with chronic pain, as I have outlined frequently, your whole life gets flipped upside down. But, having goals to work towards, can improve your overall mindset, and really boost your morale.

Now goal setting may seem like something an 80-year-old therapist may recommend. Everyone has heard of the strategy most likely, but there is a certain way to structure goal setting to make the most of the practice, and make it seem less mundane, and less of a chore.

Some people when they set goals, they make them quite large, sometimes unattainable, and sometimes very far off in the future. Examples of this can include they want to be an entrepreneurial billionaire, they want to own a mansion, they want to be a fitness model with the perfect body. Now these are all fine goals to have, but you will notice that these are quite rare feats. If these are your goals, you are setting yourself up for failure because the chances of succeeding are quite low. There are not that many billionaires, and the fitness industry is saturated with people who want to be fitness models, and achieving the perfect body is something most don't achieve as even if you look great you will always find things you want to improve upon.  These goals listed also take time, years, maybe even decades to achieve if ever. After a certain amount of time it is so common to abandon the goal if the result seems so out of reach.

The key I learned is balance. You want to have both short-term goals and long-term goals. What I found helpful was that you make only a few long-term goals. By long term I mean that it will take at least a year to achieve if not longer. These long-term goals should be goals that you can accomplish with hard work and are achievable. But we also want to make smaller goals that in the end will help us achieve our bigger goals. These smaller goals are ones that we can accomplish every day, or every week.

To give you a better understanding of what I am talking about let's dive into a goal that I made for myself. My number one goal for a long time throughout this journey was heading back to work and starting my career in the criminal justice field. This may seem like a simple goal to have for the average person, but for me it was not. With the symptoms I had on a regular basis, holding a normal job was impossible.

Having shifts every day, a regular schedule, doing all the necessary duties one does in a day of work, was something that I could not do. I made it one of my long-term goals because it seemed far off for where I was both mentally and physically. I knew it was something that eventually should be achievable, but that I was going to have to put in a lot of work to be able to do. I made it a long-term goal because of all the things having a career brings you. First, an income in which you can live independently and have your own place. An income that gives you freedom to travel where you like; there are so many places in the world I want to visit. And finally, a sense of purpose; it has always been my dream to have a career where I can help people.

But from where I started, how was I going to achieve this long-term goal of mine? I first had to make several short-term goals, things I could do every day, which would help me reach this long-term goal of mine. I made a list of activities that I wanted to do throughout the day to help me physically. This included training, physiotherapy, walking, stretching, foam rolling, breathing exercises, light weights, and reaching certain number of steps walked every day. For the average person, these may not even seem like goals, just something that could be accomplished in a couple hours. But for me, they were challenging. Next, I made a list of activities that would help me mentally. This included meditation, staying off my phone and social media, and using the many coping mechanisms for pain outlined earlier.

All these activities were made into a check list on my phone. These are goals and activities that I wanted to achieve every day, and while I did them, I would check them off. I would make sure that I did not go through a day without doing them, because I knew if I did, it would set me back. Procrastination would set in, and one day without doing them could turn into weeks, or months. Every day that I accomplished these, seemed like a small victory, and made me feel good about myself. Of course there were hard days in which there was no way that I could do all or even any of these things, but having terrible days was out of my control, and I had to cut myself some slack when this happened. What I think is also important is to write these goals down. Have them viewable, so you see them every day, and you are reminded of them, and what you are working towards.

I also had other goals, but they were ones that I could do when the time was right, and I was feeling okay. These I called mid-term goals. Some of these included going to a hockey game, going out for beer and wings at a pub, going for a hike in the mountains, playing golf, playing tennis, visiting my best friend in Edmonton, going back to work at my old produce job. Some of these were activities that for many years I could not do at all, or if I could, it was hard and rare. But slowly as I started having some better days, I realized that they could be achieved. As I started to be able to check some of these off my list, I added new activities that would push me even more, and added other things that I haven't been able to do for a long time. Now, something as simple as going out for wings at a restaurant is something, I can do the majority of days without thinking about it, when before, my symptoms wouldn't allow it as the environment would be excruciating. That lets me know that my hard work is slowly paying off.

So, there was an example for me. You had one long term goal, you had many short-term daily goals, and you had mid-term goals. Working every day at the short-term goals helped me achieve the mid-term goals that I had set. The more mid-term goals I checked off, the closer I felt towards reaching my long-term goal.

Goal setting has several benefits, but you will only notice them if you really stick with it. You must ask yourself what is it that I really want to accomplish in my life. What is important to me? And what am I doing to try to achieve these things?  Having a structured plan in place, where you outline what your goals are, and how you are going to achieve them, makes it much more likely that you will succeed.

# Chapter 17:

## Confidence

One of the reasons I felt compelled to write about goal setting is that it segues into my next topic, which is about confidence. Of course one of the main reasons for goal setting is a way to beat procrastination, and ultimately get things done, but as an added bonus, every time you complete a goal, no matter if it's a small, medium, or large one, it gives you confidence. It makes you feel good about yourself.

Chronic pain wears on you mentally so much, that often you will start to question yourself, question if you can do things, question if doing an activity might make your symptoms worse. Every day that we fight back against this mentality, and complete our goals, we are gaining confidence inourselves.

I believe a lot of the confidence we have in ourselves as an adult, starts at an early age. If you were a kid like me, who was constantly bullied and made fun of, those effects sometimes can last a lifetime. As I mentioned earlier, the bullying really took its toll on my confidence, affecting me for years. If I did not have the self-awareness to try to change how I felt about myself through hard work, I still may be feeling very bad about myself. On the contrary, if you grew up being popular, on all the sports teams, never having troubles making friends and never being bullied, having confidence in yourself may never be a problem in your life.

But what does confidence have to do with dealing with chronic pain?

When my first symptoms started, as I wrote in my story, it was brushed off by my doctor as anxiety. And even though I did not think he was correct, I figured he knew me very well, and that maybe he was right and maybe the medication he was pushing would help me. Even though I outlined all the symptoms that I was going through, I did not stand up for myself when he labeled what I had as just a mental illness. I questioned myself. Maybe I was just going crazy or something, since basic initial testing showed that nothing should be wrong with me that would explain my symptoms. This made me feel less inclined to seek other opinions. I did not want to hear that it was all just anxiety from another doctor. I did not want to hear that I was fine when I felt I was not.

As my symptoms progressed, doctors and specialists that I saw just wanted to throw certain medications at me and see what stuck. It felt like I was not being taken seriously, and it felt like they truly thought I was exaggerating when I told them my symptoms. Everybody I saw came up with only band-aid solutions, or dismissed me, not how we could get to the root of the problem and fix it.

What I learned was that I was being too passive when going to my appointments. I was joking around, laughing with my doctors, as I do with everybody, and thus I believe, was not taken as seriously as I should have been. I did not have the confidence to really stand up for myself. Little did they know, most of the time I was crying my eyes out before and after the appointment for how bad I felt, and I sucked it up and put on a brave face when I went in.

Things started to change when I did my own research on what was going on with me; when I started getting second, third, and fourth opinions; when I strongly urged my doctors to send me to specialists when they were on the fence about it. The more knowledge I gained about my situation, the more I was able to engage with people about what was going on and realize if this person could help me or not. I was the one, through my own research, that found out what was the root problem of my pain and symptoms. I was the one who found the right doctors, specialists, surgeons, and physios to see that could help me. I started to speak up for myself when I felt I had to, and that's when things started to get done.

Had I had the confidence in myself early on to speak up, perhaps things would have gotten caught earlier. Perhaps I would be much further along than I am now, and there would have been less complications. But I cannot go back in time, I can only learn from the experience. I can only look at the positive side, in that I am happy that I eventually did stand up for myself and do my own research. If I had not, I still may be dealing with severe symptoms and thinking that I am crazy.

So many people over the years have messaged me saying they have had similar experiences in both people and doctors brushing them off and not being taken seriously. For many, and like myself, it is the frustrations that come with having an "invisible illness". This is when your symptoms are not obvious to anyone on the outside, where as, say you are in a wheelchair with a cast, which is quite obvious. It is hard to put into words what having an invisible illness feels like to a normal person, but, since you have learned how great at analogies I am, I will try. It is almost like your leg is broken and you are in a cast, but you have people constantly telling you, you are fine, keep walking on that leg. There is nothing wrong, it is not broken it is all in your head, you look okay to me. Clearly you know that your leg is broken, that you should not be walking on it, that you are in crazy amounts of pain, but no one can tell, but you.

I had a great amount of frustration early on when no one could tell just how I was feeling. No one could see the amount of pain I was in, no one could see how nauseous I was unless I was throwing up, no one could tell how dizzy I was, and when I developed PTSD, no one could see all the symptoms associated with that. But, through all the coping mechanisms I have learned over the years, as well as sticking up for myself and getting to the root cause of my problems, I have gained confidence in myself. Confidence has made it easier to get up in the morning and say to myself, this is what I have, this is what

I'm going through, this is who I am and that is okay. It has made interactions with others easier. You may not be able to see my symptoms, see how bad I feel, but that is okay. Confidence has as well made it easier to drown out the outside world, and focus on myself, on getting better, and not feel bad for being selfish about it.

# Chapter 18:

## Where to Start?

Now that I have outlined some of my strategies for dealing with chronic pain mentally, it may seem like a daunting task on where to start if you are dealing with your own chronic issues. It may feel like everyone is trying to give you advice, trying to help you, but how do I begin to implement all these changes in my life. And if I do, am I doing enough? Or too much? It is so common to be overwhelmed on where to begin and these thoughts are very normal when trying to make changes in your life. It is human nature to second guess yourself or be unsure about a new path or direction in your life. Change does not come overnight; it takes time to see results, and it takes time to see the payoff. You must put in the work.

Changing the way, you think can be a monumental task, and it is not a bad thing if you have to ask for outside help to guide you. As I wrote before, I saw a psychologist that really helped me on my journey, and helped me quite a bit with coping strategies, and turning my mind into a not so scary place. There's nothing wrong with seeking out someone that may help you, and you may have to go through a few psychologists or therapists until you find one that works for you, but it can make a world of difference. As I mentioned, for me, she was there to listen, and help me reframe my thoughts. She was there to guide me, give me a gentle push when I needed it, motivate me, and give me confidence. The more open and honest I was with her, and the more work that I put in, the more benefits I received back.

What also helped guide me was picking up a self-help book. At first mention of a self-help book you may get frightened away and scoff at the idea, but in all honesty these books can be a useful tool for anybody. A lot of them are very well written, full of knowledge and insight, and really speaks to the human condition. You do not need chronic pain, illness, depression, or anxiety to get benefits. The books I found most useful were ones that were part book, part workbook, where you can write inside the book when they give you exercises or tasks. I found this balance of both was helpful as just reading a lot of information often is not that supportive to making a lasting change in your life. It can be boring and uninspiring. But if you combine this information and knowledge with the workbook aspect, doing activities and exercises, it really engages you, and reinforces the information in a personal way.

A lot of these books emphasize cognitive behavioural therapy, teaching you, and making you aware of thoughts, behaviours, and actions that you may be doing that is harmful towards your mental health. CBT is a lot about analyzing your own thoughts and keeping track of what you are thinking about. Writing down these thoughts that you are having, the thoughts that give you anxiety or the thoughts that make you depressed or bring fear. Once written down, you go through them and ask yourself if these thoughts have any truth to them, or are they just manifestations of your mind, where you are over thinking and catastrophic thinking. All of us at some point over think and have untrue thoughts, so it is very common. But instead of trying to eliminate these thoughts, you must frame them into something that is not harmful to your mind.

For example, let's say you are analyzing thoughts that you are having about going to the doctor on Friday. You are a nervous person, and you are quite scared of going. Your thoughts may include that, "I won't be able to go because I'll be feeling really sick from being anxious, or that if I do go I will make a fool or myself because I won't know what to say and I will look stupid and the doctor will think I'm stupid. Maybe they will find something wrong with me like cancer, and I rather not know about it. Or maybe they will find nothing, and the doctor will think I am crazy, and maybe I am crazy."

Once you go through and analyze these thoughts, you start to realize how untrue and unrealistic they are. You realize okay how many doctors' appointments have I been to? Probably dozens. Of these dozens of appointments how many did you miss because you were so anxious. Okay, you have not missed any appointments. How many times did you go where you felt like you made a fool of yourself and looked stupid?  I do not think that has happened before; it is turned out okay every time you have gone. How likely is it that they will find something as serious as cancer? Very low. So, when you sit back after analyzing the thoughts you realize that everything that you were thinking of is a worst-case scenario, or things that have never happened before. You have convinced yourself how horrible it is going to be, but every time you have gone to the doctors it has turned out fine and made it through it with no problems.

After doing this exercise repeatedly, it will start to show you that your patterns of thought are wrong, and you will learn to reframe these thoughts. You will instead think, okay I am feeling anxious about this appointment, but I have been to lots of other ones before and nothing bad happened, and nothing bad will happen this time either. It will go well just like all the other appointments and I will make it through just like I have every time before. Over time you are convincing and retraining your brain, and it is not even convincing, it is the actual truth. Over time you will start to get less anxious about situations that usually had brought on anxiety before. You will start to have less fear and have more confidence in yourself.

There are so many other aspects of CBT, but essentially, you are retraining yourself to think rationally, properly, and truthfully. When we do not, we create all sorts of thoughts in our minds that give us fear, anxiety, depression, which can bring out emotions and behaviours that can hinder our everyday lives. These workbooks are a great tool to guide you through the process of understanding yourself and making you more self-aware.

Another good starting block is to be open and honest with a close friend or loved one. If you are going through a hard time, tell them, explain the thoughts you are having, what you are feeling, and everything that is going on. Finding someone close to do this with can be hard, but hopefully we all have at least one person we feel comfortable opening up to. This can make a huge difference on several levels. Having someone even just to listen can be a huge relief, but often times they will have advice, or have gone through similar things, making you feel less alone, and perhaps being able to use their experience or advice to help you as well.

Being open and honest with someone also can allow you to form a closer bond and a closer friendship. It is very common to have drinking friends, or partying friends. People that you hang out with but only in social situations, and only to have fun. But when you sit back, do you really know a lot about them? Do you know what hardships they are going through or thoughts they may be having? Do they share personal details about themselves or open up about things?  Do they share the shame love of Vietnamese iced coffee as you?

A drinking buddy friendship can be great and obviously fun, but when the time comes and you are going through a rough time, will they be there for you? Will they have any empathy, or care? It is important to try and form at least a few close friendships where the answer to all the above questions is yes. Friendships where you do not have to go out and party, or drink, where you can literally do anything at any time, and still enjoy yourselves and have fun. It is not easy putting yourself out there, making yourself vulnerable, but most of us are in the same position, and most of us are searching for deeper connections and deeper friendships. We have more in common with each other than we think.

Starting to make changes in your life, how you think, behave, and act, is not easy. We have built up a lifetime of habits, and it can be stressful to change these. Again, it is going to be discouraging, daunting, and hard at the beginning, because you will want to see changes right away. Finding a person to help you through the journey can be a key to long-term success, as can finding resources whether it is books, online, or through classes.

<u>Chapter 19:</u>

## Other Lessons

While I have talked a lot about what I have learned on how to deal with chronic pain, what I have not dived into a lot about is what I have learned about life in general.

It was very humbling to me when all this health stuff started happening, and over the years it made me realize what is important in life. One of the things I realized is that we need to be living for ourselves. We need to be living for what makes us happy, which is different for every single person. Striving towards inner peace and acceptance, learning to love who we are, and embracing every little thing about ourselves is important. We cannot worry about the pressures of society, friends, or family. They will have their own ideas of what you should do, how you should act, who you should be. But this will mostly always differ from who you really are.

The pursuit of money is not everything in life, and I think too many people get fixated on every little detail of their finances, or how much things cost. Of course, everyone needs money to survive. We need food, shelter, water, clothing, and all of that. But our basic needs are as easily attainable now, as they were in any point in history. For almost the entire time man has been on the Earth, he has spent his whole day trying to achieve these things. It took a whole day just tracking down an animal for food; a stream for water; collecting wood for shelter and warmth. We do not need to do any of those things anymore. Everything we need to survive is easily accessible. But society has ingrained in us that we need more to be happy. We need a nicer house, a better car, expensive electronics, a beanie baby collection, and if we do not, we will be looked down upon, seen as unsuccessful. But these things do not make us happy; they just fill whatever void we have, until it is time to make the next purchase to distract ourselves.

It is not money that is the most important thing; it is the experiences that we have in life.  It is also the people that we have these experiences with. During my most difficult days, I did not think back to the nice things that I bought myself over the years, or the superficial purchases that I made. Although I love my stereo system, I thought back to all the memories that I had over the years with my friends and family. All the trips I took and all the adventures that I went on. All the nights staying up talking and laughing. This is what I remembered during my darkest times, and that brought a smile to my face, and joy in my heart.

Finding friendships that are meaningful and finding people to share life with makes the experiences that you have even more special. From personal experience, it seems a lot of time once someone finds a significant other, they often neglect or abandon a lot of the friendships that they had before. They do not put in as much effort or make time to talk to their friends on a regular basis. I understand that as we get older, we have more commitments and less free time, but it is all about what you make a priority. Even something as simple as a phone call to a friend, can really have a positive impact on not only their life, but yours as well.

<u>Chapter 20:</u>

## Divisiveness

Another thing I have learned is not to buy into the divisiveness that society seems to be headed into or has been for several years. It seems everybody is against somebody. Liberals vs. conservatives. Religious vs. nonreligious. Men vs. women. Old vs. young. Caucasian vs. minorities. And of course, the endless propaganda, fake news, and similar rhetoric that is happening.

Because of the nature of my work, promotion of my business is a big aspect, and the majority of this is being done on social media. But social media has changed. It is less about connecting with your friends, and more about sharing videos, news articles, memes, etc. A lot of these are biased towards one side or another, usually devoid of any facts, and in comment sections, there is much hatred towards almost anything or anyone.

With the ever expansion of the internet, it has allowed those who share a common view, however obscure it may be, to come together. When this happens, people feel like they belong and have a voice, but on the other hand, it festers what hatred they might have, and closes their mind off to any other views and opinions. This hatred has obviously even been spilled offline, with people being more brazen and outspoken in public. Obviously, freedom of speech is important, but not when its hate filled.

To me, this is all saddening to see, especially watching people I once knew very well fall into the trap and become very angry at the world and certain people. I think its important to remember that everybody has a different view of the world. Everyone has experienced different things in their life and has had a different upbringing. How you were raised, what your education was, where you lived, what your religion may or may not be, shapes your views, and shapes you into the person that you are today. But just because someone's view is different than yours does not mean they are wrong, or stupid. Everyone has a different opinion on what matters to them in life.

The best thing we can do is inform ourselves, and form our own opinions, not from what someone tells us to. If you are into politics, research the positions that the political parties have on certain issues, especially issues that are important to you. Research the candidates themselves that you are choosing from. Politics should not be a "team" thing like sports, where you blindly support a party or candidate no matter what. Parties change, their views change, as do the people who run them. While doing your own research you may be surprised that the party or candidate you support, does not share the same views or values that you do. Elections have real consequences, and there is no excuse not to vote, or not to know anything about who or what you are voting for.

We are all in this together is a common saying, and one that I agree with. Nobody truly knows what I have been through in my life. But I also do not know what other people have been through either. So, if someone has a different view than I do, I try to be understanding, and compassionate, and try to remember that it is okay not to agree with someone. I also try to remember that it is good to form relationships with others who are outside our normal social circles. Some of my best friendships are from people with different ethnic backgrounds, different religious backgrounds, and different upbringings. Its refreshing to learn their perspectives, and even helps me learn and grow as a person, to see life and the world from a different angle. When we foster acceptance instead of hate, we draw people towards us in a friendly manner, instead of pushing people away.

# Chapter 21:

## Physical

This part of the book is about the physical things I have done, or treatments that I have had, that have worked for me. As you can imagine, having dealt with what I have been for over 7 years, I have seen my fair share of people from all sorts of different fields. As my case was unique, initially it was hard to find the right people and the right treatments. But I never gave up my search and kept on fighting to find any sort of relief. As most people are aware of the basic treatments for chronic pain, I wanted to outline treatments that really helped me, but that are not common knowledge to many people. Thankfully, these therapists and practitioners I saw agreed to help me, and explain these treatments in their own words, because who better to help you understand just what it is they do. I included these treatments in the first part of the book, and they are again, NUCCA chiropractic care, functional patterns training, and myofunctional therapy. If any of these treatments speak to you, and seem like they might be able to help, I urge you to look into it even more, and find someone in your city that will be able to help you.

I have been asked numerous times about other tips or advice. For a lot of you with chronic pain or illness, lots of these will be things others have suggested trying numerous times, I am sure.

First, I cannot recommend any sort of prescription medication. What I have learned over the years is that everybody is completely different, and what may help me, may make you feel much worse, or visa versa. There are so many different medications in the chronic pain world, in the migraine world, and even some for vertigo, nausea, etc. The best advice I can give you is to follow the advice of your doctors. As much as It seems that I have had a bad experience with them, they usually have been on the ball in terms of knowledge and willingness to try different drugs. These doctors will know better than anyone what drugs may help subside some symptoms, but ultimately it is up to you to do a trial and error to see if they will help you. Always remember that with a lot of drugs, there will be side effects, so you will have to weigh the pros and cons of taking them. Throughout the years I have tried dozens of different things, but as mentioned earlier, felt the best taking nothing at all. Today, all I take is a low dose of a medication intended for nerve pain. This medication helps me, the only downside is it makes me quite tired.

Closely related to prescriptions, I have had many people ask about supplements, and I give almost the same answer. There are tons of different supplements available, and tons of different brands. Again, what may work for you, may not work for me. Just remember that the supplement market is unregulated, and often you do not know the purity of what you are getting. As well, supplements can be expensive, and are not covered, so you will have to weigh the risk of cost vs. benefit. Always remember to check if a certain supplement may interact badly with a medication that you are on. I have not had any significant result with supplements, and again have probably tried dozens. I do not regularly take anything, other than the occasional multi vitamin.

Diet is important yes. And like medications and supplements, everybody is different. Everybody reacts to foods differently. I believe eating healthy is one of the best things that we can do for ourselves. I am not going to promote a certain diet, or certain foods, but I would strongly encourage anyone to both enjoy food but be smart about serving size. For myself, many different diets were recommended to try to alleviate inflammation and pain, but none seemed to have any effect. I even got a food sensitivity test to see what foods I seem to react to. These foods included, milk of every kind, grains of every kind, gluten free grains of every kind, various types of legumes, various types of nuts, and funny enough, oranges. I cut out these foods out of my diet for a long time, which was hard, but had no results. Today, I will not say no to any types of food, including those high on my sensitivity list, I just make sure that my portion size is not large. I try eating as many fresh fruits and vegetables as I can, as well as lean meats. I believe that good food is one of the treasures of life, and I always look forward to trying something new.  Cannot forget about my shrimp too!

One of the butting jokes of those of us in the chronic illness community is that it seems the most common advice given to us is make sure that you are drinking enough water. I won't say much more than that about water, but yes, it is important to make sure you are getting enough, especially if you have chronic pain/illness, and especially if you are taking medications and supplements. Staying properly hydrated is one of the easiest things we can do, and one of the most beneficial as well.

Exercise is another topic that gets brought up frequently. Again, I do not need to go into a big explanation of how important exercise is, because we are all aware of it. But what I think is important is to get as much exercise outside as possible when you can, as opposed to at the gym, or inside. Also, I think its important to tailor exercise around your limitations, if you have any, and find activities that you can do that do not bring about great stress to your body. Exercise should not end with grade 12 gym class, and like eating healthy, staying active is one of the best things we can do for ourselves. Even going out for a walk everyday is something so simple, but so beneficial.

Sleep is also another topic that most of us are now aware plays a very important role in our lives. For those of us who suffer from chronic pain/illness, getting a proper sleep can seem impossible, and only exacerbate any issues we might have. Like many experts say, getting at least 8 hours is important, but what is equally as important is your time leading up to going to sleep. Staying off electronics, staying away from bright lights, avoiding eating big meals and exercise, are all things we should be doing a couple hours leading up to sleep. As well, activities such as reading, listening to music, meditating, stretching, are all good activities to calm us down, and get us ready for sleep. Having the correct pillow can also make a huge difference, and it is important to find one that is both supportive, and comfortable. My house is littered with a dozen pillows that I have tried over the years, safe to say I have enough to build a fort or two.

Most of you will be familiar with seeing a physiotherapist, massage therapist, and chiropractor, however, not all are made equal, and it is important to find ones that can help you and make a difference, and not just drain your wallet. I saw several physiotherapists over the years, and on a whole, I loved getting to know, talking, and spending time with them. However, as much as I liked them, I saw little to no progress or results. Because of this, I had to keep searching, and thankfully I ended up finding both Naurine for myofunctional therapy, and Ben for basically everything else using Functional Patters. It was so discouraging to feel like I had wasted time, effort, and money with no results, and if you feel the same, I encourage you to still do your research, ask around, and try multiple practitioners until you find someone and something that helps.

Similarly, it took a long time to finally find a massage therapist that really made a difference. Again, over the years I met a number of them that I liked, but none that made a significant difference with the number of knots and muscle issues I was having. Thankfully a few years into my journey, I did find one, and he was amazing at not only breaking up the huge knots I had all over my body, but also breaking up scar tissue that had formed through various injuries and surgeries. Sometimes, massages are not meant to be relaxing and peaceful. What worked for me was deep tissue, and if you have ever had it done, it can be very unpleasant, and even painful. I as well have been seeing a cranio sacral therapist for many years. Instead of targeting muscles, these therapist work on the facia of the body. It is much lighter than a massage, and different, but still effective for many people, including myself.

Chiropractic care helped me a lot, but only after a few trial and errors. I loved the chiro's that I saw before I met Dr. Abreu, but the relief was either too short lived, or none at all. Dr. Abreu's specific method of chiropractic care worked for me, and I was glad to find something that provided lasting relief.

Since the beginning of my journey, I have seen a doctor for trigger point injections, and dry needling, and I do recommend this if you have issues with muscle knots, or constantly tight muscles. It can complement any sort of physio, massage, or chiropractic care that you might be getting. This doctor, or therapist will work with you to find problem muscles that may be causing issues and using a small needle with or without a freezing agent, pierce the muscle. If injecting with a freezing agent, the needle will quickly be removed, if a dry needle, the needle will be left in for usually around 10 minutes. This relaxes the muscle, and if the needle is inserted in the right place, help to break up any knots.

Of course, with all these practitioners I saw, I as well saw dozens more different doctors, or specialists, or surgeons. But I saw these professionals because they tailored to what I was going through. Like I mentioned earlier, if you are going through something, please do your own research, talk to your doctor, a second doctor, a third doctor, however many doctors you feel you need, to solve an issue if you are having one. Do not leave any stone unturned.

Lastly, I am a big believer in light therapy. Sadly, not of the disco ball variety. You may have noticed that I have wrote encouraging being outside a lot, and one of the biggest reasons for that, is the benefits that the sun has. It plays a crucial role in how our bodies function, and of course gives us vitamin D. Most of us who live in colder climates will be deficient. But what do we do when its wintertime, and the sun sometimes does not shine, or is very weak? I ended up buying something called a "happy light." It tricks the brain and body into thinking that it is actually the sun, minus the UV rays. This light therapy is best used in the morning, shone on the face, as the main function is to reset the bodies circadian rhythm. I noticed feeling better in the morning with more energy, and feeling more tired at bedtime, and easier to sleep.

The other light therapy I use, is red light therapy. This is a device that uses both a red light, and infrared light, which you shine onto your face or your body. This type of therapy used to be only common in spas, as they were quite expensive. Nowadays, you can get your hands on a small one for a reasonable price, but just be sure that you are buying from a reputable source, as they are easy to fake. The benefits to red light therapy are many, and it is probably best you look them up. In short, it has shown to decrease inflammation, and increase blood flow, when shone on a given area. I mostly use this on my head and neck, and most often it decreases whatever pain or headache that I am having at the time.

Just remember that anything physical to help with chronic pain or illness will be a trial and error. Make sure you give a certain practitioner, therapy, medication, or supplement enough of a chance to work. This can often be weeks, and there often can be side effects, before starting to work. As I mentioned before, it is crucial to remember that everyone is different, everyone will respond differently to different therapies.

<u>Part 3: An Outsiders Perspective</u>

## Chapter 22: Perspective "A"

In my book, I really thought it was important to get a 360-degree scope of chronic illness and pain. Obviously, I wanted to give you my perspective, what I went through, what I learned, what helped me etc. But what often gets missed or overlooked is just how chronic conditions affect those around the sufferer as well. I thought it was important for the closest to me, to write about their experience. I asked three of them to each write a small section for me. But I did not want them to write about me specifically. I did not want them to write about praising me, or if they felt bad for me, etc. (They of course broke this rule, haha) I wanted them to truly show their feelings about what they went through.

Because chronic issues so greatly impacts those closest to the sufferer, that they almost are suffering along with me at times. I wanted them to write about their perspective, what they learned, what they went through, and how this all impacted them. So, if it seems like they are being selfish at times and writing all about themselves, it is because I asked them to! Thankfully, the perspectives are all different. I have a perspective from both genders, perspectives of friends that knew me before my chronic issues, and perspectives of one that I met in the midst of all this, who never knew me before this all started. I gave them each a rough outline of what I wanted them to write about and let them take it from there. One of them left some of the questions in their write up, and as I did not want to disturb or change at all what they had wrote, I left it unedited.  Here is the first perspective, "A"

"I have known Ryan for about 20 years, since we were 10 years old. Initially we knew each other through playing sports, but our friendship really grew in high school, when we finally went to the same school as each other. We had a mutual group of friends that we hung out with in, and outside of school, and so many good times were had. Unfortunately, after high school, my family decided to move back to my hometown, about 3 hours away. However, moving away did not dampen our friendship, it seemed to make it even stronger. Over the next few years after high school, we formed such a close, special. and important bond. We visited each other multiple times a year while we were both in university, having some of the best times of our lives. However, this got abruptly interrupted by, as you have read by now, Ryan's health issues.

**When this whole ordeal started for Ryan, what were your initial thoughts or impressions? And how has this changed overtime?**

When Ryan first began experiencing symptoms, I remember thinking this would be a minor setback for him, and it would not be long before he returned to the light-hearted, hilarious friend I could go back to adventuring with. Back then I had no experience of anyone our age seriously struggling with their health, let alone suffering from the chronic disease and setbacks that would follow in the coming years for him. Even as his closest friend, I didn't worry about his condition early on because I didn't know any better, it wasn't something young people went through and there wasn't a clear diagnosis to even know what to worry about. It seemed like a tribulation he would move past with the right medical care, treatments, and support. Looking back, I was completely wrong. This has been so much longer and painful for him than anyone would have believed.

One reason I did not see Ryan's struggles coming was because I lived in a different city. The distance made it more difficult to understand what was truly going on with him. Despite always staying in touch and sharing what is going on with our lives, words do not always do justice to people's suffering. I don't think it's how our emotions work, sometimes we have to see and feel what someone is going through to get a sense of their struggle and speak directly to express our emotion whether it's pain or joy. Only after seeing him suffer on his hard days and listening to him describe his suffering did I start to feel the weight of it. It is important to spend quality time with someone to really grasp how their feeling, otherwise it may not sink in.

Another reason I did not panic was because of the uncertainty around Ryan's diagnosis, which probably sounds strange. The constellation of mental and physical symptoms he experienced did not fit neatly into any label doctors could identify, and if doctors did not have a reason to be worried, I didn't think I should have one either. Doctors are people who spend lives understanding the human body and mind, people we trust to give us sound advice about our health. Looking back, Ryan was misled by many medical professionals and his suffering was made worse by their incompetence. It is one thing to not be able to figure out the medical issue, but it is another to push a person down the wrong path and cause potentially more suffering. In many cases, more harm was done than good for Ryan.

But if a doctor does not know what is happening, how is anyone else supposed to know how to react? When someone tells you they have cancer, we all understand what that means. When it's unclear what someone is dealing with, you don't know how to behave around them, what to say to make it better if it even gets better, or how to explain their suffering to other people. Some people even believe you might be faking it. Ryan's diagnosis never came with an instruction manual, he has had to do his own research, double-check professionals, and pursue alternative help as well.

Like some of the medical advice he received, I hoped it was a simple issue or that it would resolve itself with rest and some care. I know he had to justify his health issues to others for a long time because people were suspicious or minimized his suffering thinking it would just pass and it's clear to me why he had to do that now. Never for a moment did I believe he was faking the pain, headaches, and symptoms. I just did not have a way to understand his experience early on and I think many people in his life came from that confused place.

Once his symptoms began to worsen a couple years into his journey and he had seen multiple specialists without hearing any real answers, I started to worry. That worrying that has not stopped since. There were moments where I thought he may finally round the corner when he had many good days in a row, and others I thought he may want to end his life with constant up and downs like this. I worry I may lose my friend to this or even if he is alive just seeing his spirit shattered is a form of death in its own way too. At times I am gloomy about whether he is ever going to make it out of this, but in my heart, I choose to believe he is going to come out as healthy as he went in.

I believe this because I desperately want my friend back, and want him to experience the life he deserves, the life I have.

From thinking it was purely his severely misaligned jaw, concussions, and nerve damage, to Lyme Disease and body misalignment, it has been an emotional ride and an education for everybody in Ryan's close circle. So yes, things have changed a lot from when he first got sick. I went from not knowing how to relate to Ryan's experience to just wishing I could take it all away from him when you see the life he has to live on terrible days. Life really puts a burden on people who are chronically ill, not just with dealing with their issue, but having to handle their illness in their social life and explain their suffering. It's hard enough feeling severe pain in your body, but to explain it and turn away people in your life because you can't maintain relationships is an extra layer of suffering, I had never thought about. It is terrible.

**What have you learned from being friends with someone in chronic pain? As well, how has it impacted your own life or your views?**

It is hard to put into words everything Ryan has taught me. What I can say is being a part of his life, seeing what he has gone through and how he has responded has made me a more appreciative and empathetic person. I am not as quick to judge someone's situation from the outside, if you look at Ryan you have no idea what he has been through and this applies to everyone. While I wish his journey could have been different, even Ryan would tell you he is grown into a stronger person having gone through this hell. His will to find happiness in his suffering is a reminder of how precious my moments are and how much better I can be to the people around me while I have a healthy mind and body.

 Being the humble guy he is, he will also tell you that anyone in his position would rise to the occasion like him, but in my experience, adversity does not push everyone to be better. In fact, it destroys many people's lives, but it made him even better. He finds a way to smile in the face of excruciating pain that is relentless for days, pull positivity from so many hopeless and dizzying moments, commit to hours of physiotherapy and meditation exercises, and *still* create opportunities for himself through painting, social media, and now with this book that I feel very fortunate to write words for. He is so grateful for the opportunity to just experience life symptom free. Seeing this rewires your own brain to recognize what is important. It is about the people on this ride with you, not the other distractions we easily get caught in. When he is feeling well, he does not need any reason outside of himself to just be happy with what he has right here right now. Many people spend their healthy life being miserable, chasing expectations of what their life should look like rather than enjoying the place it is actually in. I fall into this trap at times, but I often pull myself out quicker when I think of Ryan. When I am struggling or feeling exhausted, I think of what he has been through and find strength to give more to what I care about. It does not always work, but you must make the effort and strive in your life for better.

Seeing these things play out in him forced me to find joy in simple things too, which I was not used to and often struggled with. He helped me see happiness can be found by just existing, where I can look back and see all the moments, I created my own problem. He is so happy to just spend time and talk or shoot some hoops, I can feel it off him. The gratitude to connect just pours out of him over these simple things. It becomes harder to take your excuses seriously when you're friends with someone suffering from chronic health issues. In some ways, he helped strip away the games I play that keep me from being happy whether it is pursuing my real passions, being vulnerable with others, or taking real risks in life. What do I really have to lose? He is fighting for such basic parts of his life sometimes while I get to entertain these higher-level fears around who I am and what I want out of life. It does not mean I should not worry, but they hold a little less weight when I check in to see how Ryan is doing. If you are not careful, your mind will try to generate problems in your life, especially when things are going well, and this is something I watch out for now. Ryan does not have to worry about that he has plenty of issues to tackle. When we go through conflict, life will strip away these mental games to let us pursue what we want with more tenacity and appreciation. On Ryan's good days he wants to conquer the world and I try to borrow this mentality as much as I can.

He has also forced me to ask questions to myself that are hard to confront. Truly, who are we to say our health does not come to a screeching halt tomorrow? No one plans to get sick or suffer. Did I soak in the good days with laughter or let the small annoyances bring me down? Did I experience life, or did I sit on the sidelines of the adventure in fear? Did I work hard, and realize the potential I have in myself and offer it to others? Did I really share myself with friends, family, lovers or even strangers and make their lives immeasurably better? I keep these questions close to heart thanks to Ryan, and he motivates me to answer them better. He is helped me live in a way that aligns with better answers, ones that are truer to who I am deep down even though I still have a lot of work to do. We talked about these questions more when life started to pose them to us earlier than others in our social circle. Now we push one another to be better, can cry when things look helpless and help one another see our lives and relationships more clearly.

When I look back, these big questions led me to pursue a new career, move to New York, fall in love, experiment with teaching, improv, yoga, meditation, confront my own social anxiety, and build new friendships as well. Of course, these things would have been better with Ryan on the journey, but he was always on my mind as I moved through them. These are also questions some people start asking too late or never come to accept inside themselves, but they came early for us and I am grateful for that. Throughout the wild journey that was my 20's not once did Ryan ever ask me to stop living my life either. He knew and told me I should be out exploring, and I still hope we can do that together down the road.

For most of our 20's, Ryan and I lived extremely different lives but still maintained such a strong friendship. I think it just speaks to how well we know each other, and the effort we invest to continue to grow together in all these small ways. It is easier to be brave when you have someone in your life that knows you to your core and accepts you the same after your utter failures and embarrassments. I think our relationship has helped us both stare down fear, and the possibility of failure when we brush up against hard times because we know each other's deepest worries and problems. The adversity he's faced has only brought us closer together and it's opened my eyes to the suffering others face in his position, that being a true friend is how you treat a person in times of struggle, that being emotionally vulnerable is the foundation of all relationships. Another interesting thing I have noticed is I believe many male relationships are emotionally stunted. Watching Ryan suffer forced us to bond in ways that are different than most of my other male friendships because you cannot help but feel the pain along with him. We were always on the more sensitive side, but I think those qualities helped us form a deeper relationship where we could explore our issues and not feel judged too. Take it from me, that is so rare in male relationships and I know we are both so grateful to have that. I know it has helped us both get through hard times, and it feels great to know you really understand a person and they see you clearly.

I am big believer that adversity brings out the best in us, and Ryan is one of the most extreme examples I can think of. It might feel like he would have been this other person if not for the illness, but I see at is the illness only brought out more of the great character that was inside him already. Difficulties just expose who we are, and we all have great qualities in us worth cultivating through these hard times. While I do not seek out pain, I try to embrace adversity with the same strength he brings to his own battles each day. These are also some of the benefits of being his friend beyond the laughs, love and support we offer to each other. Problems are in your way for a reason, they will make you better if you embrace them! I've learned a lot from him and couldn't convey all of it here, but if there's a takeaway it's that supporting a person suffering can mean the world to them, and open your mind to many areas of your own life you might normally look past. Being Ryan's friend will always be a good thing in my life no matter what happens.

**What are some of the greatest challenges or frustrations of being friends with someone in chronic pain?**

**What are some of the benefits of being friends with someone in chronic pain? (could be a lot of the same things as "what have you learned", but if there is any other benefits)**

The single greatest frustration of knowing someone with chronic pain is realizing you cannot have the same experiences you had with this person before their illness and being reminded of this fact repeatedly. Ryan and I went to Mexico before he was sick, partied, had plans to travel the world, broaden our social circle, maybe share an apartment. I was excited to see what shape our careers, personalities and family lives would take, and celebrate so many big milestones together. It makes me sad because these experiences feel out of reach or they are more limited due to his illness and we are not truly able to celebrate the way either of us pictured. It's hard to accept those experiences might be lost forever, especially the days where he's feeling great and you see glimpses of what you had with this person only to see it come crashing down again. I still hold out hope, but as much as I cheer him on, I also cannot count on it emotionally. There is a side seat on Ryan's rollercoaster to ride and I try to flatten it at times for my own well being. It is difficult to have your expectations set and destroyed all over again. This illness is woven into Ryan's identity, and will be around either as a symptom or a memory for the rest of his life. We all must adjust to these changes; I just want it to change in a way that is positive for him so we can seize more opportunities to enjoy no matter what form it takes. Without a doubt this is the biggest frustration.

A huge challenge you do not see until it arrives is how to grow a relationship with someone whose life no longer looks even remotely similar to yours. We first became friends because so many of our interests (ex. sports, video games, sense of humour) were the same, but for the last decade we could not have lived more differently. If there is even an ounce of disinterest in a relationship, it can drive a serious wedge between two people. We all have people that drifted away slowly who we do not speak to anymore, sometimes they live in the same city let alone far away. It is not a bad thing, it is natural as you grow through life to value different people and personalities. For some of us though a few gems stay in our lives forever. There was every reason in the world for us to drift given the circumstances.

While he was battling at home I lived on both coasts of the U.S. and Canada, taught undergraduate psychology, became an improv student, learned how to program, built new friendships, fell in and out of love many times and saw so many amazing views. I could not relate to him at all and felt guilty for sharing the fun I was having when I knew he was clinging to any shred of optimism he could find. When he can't even open his eyes without suffering, it's hard to come clean about Thursday night parties in Manhattan, deep laughs and jokes with new friends, how excited you are about the new girlfriend or getting your dream job at an amazing university. Things could not have been better for me, and things just kept getting worse for Ryan. He never made me feel bad for my own happiness and success, it was just this obvious difference that was hard to ignore whenever we spoke.

Through it all we never lost touch though, always checking in for support (yes it went both ways) and to share a few laughs (my jokes are better). As for why things did not fall apart between us; I just believe true friends know things even your partner, parents, or siblings will never get to see in you. Once you sense you know this person to their core and they genuinely feel the same, it becomes very hard to walk away from such a rare gift. Ryan's journey brought out the true colours of our friendship even more and brought us closer despite the different lives we lived.

Do I wish this person who held such a close part of my life was able to fully share it? Yes, but it was not his choice to experience this, and I do not walk away from friends in tough times. Friendship has never been more important in my life as it is now, and Ryan hammered this home for me. These are not parts of your life you can replace, they give meaning to your existence and perspective about who you really are, as well as support and sustain your well-being through the good and bad times. Deep relationships with people are everything to me, and this lesson is one benefit to being friends with Ryan.

That said, there is always a price to pay for keeping close relationships in your life and you must be ready to accept them whatever the cost may be. Ryan's health issues have been going on for over 7 years and I am so damn tired of the entire situation. It is hard to not become numb hearing the latest health issue that comes rolling in one after the another. It is not that I do not care, it is that I feel helpless to change anything, and for a long time it was only getting worse. There's nothing I can really do other than just watch my friend get hit by each wave of suffering and pain, it's been hard to accept I have no control and harder to allow myself to feel the pain of his struggles. I will often move between anger toward myself, Ryan, or the entire situation, and feeling incredibly frustrated because I cannot help but have at least some expectations of how this mess will play out. Being around Ryan and talking about it tends to awaken these expectations when he is well only to rip them to pieces when he is not feeling great. Confronting his pain is so hard that I try not to make his life harder with my disappointment, but it is also very difficult to hide and important for me to still convey where I can. It is very easy to feel numb to his experience as a means to protect yourself, feel useless or like you could be doing more.

When someone is battling chronic illness, it takes center stage in their life and will become a major part of your relationship with this person, make no mistake. It is easy for conversations to always be about health because it is their entire world, they are fighting every day. I have to say it is exhausting and frustrating to talk about health sometimes, especially when it does not feel like there is much hope of even fixing the problems and I can't even truly relate to it. It feels like an endless loop we are stuck on, where we all close our eyes, and we stumble into the exit. This can drain me because there is a never a true solution to the conversation. It has become him feeling heard by me when he explains his suffering, and the relief that comes with that. This is still important, but it is not what either of us really want to have to go through. In some ways we are just getting by, not truly fixing things or clearly moving forward. Fixing this is exactly what everyone in Ryan's life wants for him first and foremost, but people want to close this chapter for themselves as well.

No matter what happens though, the people closest to him are by his side and are not going anywhere, no matter how angry and sad they are about it. If you are going to support him on this journey you must accept that it will scar you as well. I love Ryan he will always be an important person in my life, and even if I could walk away guilt free, I would not do it. He is not a burden; he brings out my best self but if you think I am not angry with this situation you are wrong.

**From the perspective of being a friend of someone in chronic pain, is there anything else people should know?**

People need to know that someone with chronic illness will struggle to express the real level of mental or physical pain they are in all the time. You might only get a glimpse one day and another time you really see the suffering they are in because they cannot contain it anymore. It is just hard to be vulnerable and honest about setbacks all the time, but rest assured they do feel connected to you. It can be a lonely journey and it is hard to think of anything optimistic when you are in the middle of hell. As a friend or caregiver, do not take on the entire problem for the person. Just recognize you can help relieve it by supporting them with your time, attention and keeping an open mind. Feeling heard becomes everything to somebody in pain. Obviously, everyone wants to feel appreciated regardless of their health, but I think this is more pronounced when you are ill and need social connection to express your suffering. Whatever relationship you have is going to be tested through their health battle since we often learn who is truly there for us and who is not when we are struggling. It does not mean you have to be a superhero, but recognize small gestures go a long way and your support means more than they will show you most of the time."

<u>Chapter 22:</u>

## Perspective "B"

"Unfortunately, I did not know Ryan before all his pain and symptoms started. We initially met and talked online in 2016, (because millennials and crippling social anxiety and all that) and I have to say it was hands down one of the strangest encounters I have ever had with the opposite sex. I was so used to guys blowing up my phone with messages, asking to hang out, and sending unsolicited pictures, but Ryan did not do any of that. He initially seemed quite distant, uninterested, and there was barely any communication. Logically because of this, I assumed that he did not want to get to know me and was just being nice. I was always the first to message him, often asking if he wanted to come out for Taco Tuesdays at Jameson's Pub with my friends, ($5 for 3 tacos, I will take it thanks!) But he always said no, and I was always left wondering if there was something wrong with me, or that the warm welcome was finally wearing off.

One night, after getting upset at him, he finally told me a little about his medical situation, which at the time he did not have a lot of answers, only symptoms. He explained that he had severe chronic migraines which were often accompanied by vertigo, and a lot of his days were spent resting, and doing the simplest of activities. He said that he was not on his phone often, and that he was reluctant to meet me because of what he was going through.

This was laid upon me after about a month of talking on and off. In our initial conversations at the beginning he mentioned that he had some health problems, but after that, he never talked about it at all until this night. When he went into detail about what he was going through, it was hard for me to understand, let alone believe. I had never talked to anyone with health problems like he was describing. I remember I thought to myself, "Wow, what an extensive lie just to not see me, you could just tell me you are not interested." After thinking about it, and because I had nothing to lose, I called him out and told him exactly that. He was very calm about it all, and he assured me that he was not lying, and if he really did not like me, that he had no problem telling me just where I could go.

I ruminated for many days on this and decided to just go with it, he was still responding after all, and our chats were getting more frequent and going deeper than the superficial. Soon, after much persistence on my end, I asked if we could do something super simple and easy, like get a coffee at a drive thru, and sit in the car and talk afterwards. He agreed. The drive to Tim Horton's was awkward, on my end, and quiet. After we ordered and parked, we sat in silence for a bit. I was extremely shy because his pictures did not do him justice, he was freaking hot! And I had just gone through a terrible bleach job that chemically cut my beautiful curls off, and I had to rock a very unflattering bob. So, you can understand why I was feeling a bit self conscious and straight up embarrassed. This was our first time hanging out in person, and I could barely look him in the face. I sat straight, staring out the window, talking to my steering wheel the entire time. I remember him making a comment about this, and thinking it was quite funny, and my only response was to blurt out that I was just a terrible person, and that he was so good looking that it was intimidating.

We ended up talking for a few hours, about our childhood, upbringing, likes and dislikes -everything you would normally talk about when getting to know someone. He was able to explain his situation fully to me, which I still had doubts about because it seemed to unreal to have been seen by so many doctors and specialists and still not be "cured".

As time passed on, we were now beginning to hang out almost every night, as that is when his symptoms were the least severe. The more we hung out and spent time together, the harder it was for me to believe his story. Here was this seemingly normal, cute guy, talking my ear off, laughing, smiling and telling jokes, that it was hard for me to fathom the idea that he was in excruciating pain, when it did not seem like it from the outside. I kept on thinking that he could be exaggerating, and that he just suffered from bouts of migraines due to the weather or allergies, or something simple. The fact that his doctors had not found many answers was enough to keep me from believing that maybe he was stretching the truth. Nevertheless, he was one of the happiest, funny (do not tell him I said that), and most positive people I had ever met. When we were together, he made a point of never bringing how he felt into the conversation; he never once complained about his pain or fatigue. He would always try to make me laugh, and always had jokes to tell.

As time went on, I did start to believe him, as I noticed the difference in his demeanor and his mood when things were bad. I noticed a big change in his eyes, they became almost glossed over, like he was struggling to see straight. When things were bad, he struggled with even making the simplest sentences, and wherever we were, he asked if it was okay to lie down, or be in darkness. Overtime it seemed like he got more comfortable and trusted me, and he started opening a lot more about everything he had been through. Even though he was very good at explaining everything, I had a hard time comprehending it all, and it was something I struggled to completely understand.

The more time I spent with Ryan, the more I got to know him on a personal level, the more aware I became of my own biases and misconceptions towards chronic pain and illness. It was difficult for me to believe Ryan simply because he seemed okay on the outside; he was always laughing and making jokes, never taking anything seriously. I used to think to myself, "This is not that way someone acts when they are in blinding pain, it cannot be as bad as he is making it out to be." But how wrong was I! For so long I had this misconceived notion that those who had been suffering with chronic pain and illness would be bitter and wallowing in self loathing and pity, as terrible as that may sound. It was not until I met Ryan and spent time with him that he showed me just how resilient the human mind and body can be, even at its worst. Being able to see him go through all of this and still come out with a smile despite feeling like absolute hell, was truly something amazing and something to be witnessed. He also really opened my eyes to the reality of our medical system, and the many ways it fails and dismisses a lot of those with invisible illnesses and pain, just because some tests come back seemingly normal.

I never thought I would be in a situation where I would have to put myself and all my beliefs into perspective but being with Ryan has really changed a lot for me. However, I cannot say that everything was flowers and rainbows because it was not. Ryan was becoming a bigger part of my life with each passing month, but there were many things I struggled accepting and understanding with him. The big one was for a long time we rarely could do normal everyday things together. I wanted to explore the world with him, take day trips outside the city, have him meet my friends at a bar or club, go out for social gatherings. These are things that I did not think twice about, and took for granted doing, but these were things Ryan could often not do. I could not wrap my head around someone feeling so bad physically and mentally where these seemingly normal activities were so difficult. It was frustrating and something I had a very hard time with and adjusting to.

We had constant arguments about these things at first, and I could see just how difficult and crushing it was for him to say no, and to have to sit there and explain to me with tears in his eyes that he wished things could be different. I remember often thinking that he could just suck it up, and things would be okay. I was ridiculously unprepared to deal with something of this nature and being frustrated was the only emotion I often had left. I remember talking to my friends and family about him, and they constantly asked me if this was a situation I wanted to be in, and if I knew what I was getting myself into by becoming so close to someone like Ryan. It was mentally and emotionally taxing, but I cared about him so much that there was no turning back.

Ryan was extremely patient with me during this whole process of mine, more than I think I deserved. He never stopped reassuring me that my feelings were valid, and it was okay to think and feel the way I did. Looking back, I feel ashamed of my behavior and for being a bitch during such a difficult time for him. I think things really changed for me when I was able to see his daily routine firsthand, from when he first woke up, until he went to bed. In the mornings, he could barely get out of bed due to his symptoms and watching him try to get up and start his day, trying to accomplish even the smallest task lethargically really hit me hard.

I remember a specific moment, when Ryan was having a decent day, which for him was about a 7/10 pain wise. We spent the whole day outside, talking, laughing, and having the most fun. We ordered take out, and watched movies, and everything seemed to be normal. Around the middle of one of the movies, Ryan told me that he was going to lay down for a bit and grabbed an ice pack from the freezer. This was a normal occurrence as sometimes he would meditate for a bit and come back to whatever it was that we were doing. However, this time he did not come back, and some time had passed until I went to check on him and found him trying to hide his face from me. He was crying his eyes out. This was the first time I had seen him cry and things shifted into perspective for me quickly. At that moment I knew that he had been hiding how bad his pain had been throughout the day, and because of all the activities we did, it finally caught up to him. I also realized that he had been trying to down play how he was feeling a lot of the time, because he saw how difficult it had been for me to adapt to this new environment that I knew nothing about.

I felt terrible and selfish for feeling and saying the things I had complained to him so many times. Here was this amazing human who trusted me enough to show his true self to me, to let me into his chaotic life, thinking that no one would ever want to stick around knowing his situation, and being

UNDERSTANDING ABOUT MY FEELINGS - for me to complain about the most frivolous things. I cried my eyes out that night with him and apologized for my inconsiderate behavior, and he held me and had the audacity to comfort ME. Naturally this made me straight up just ugly cry into his shoulder.

For me, things were always black and white when it came to any kind of illness or pain - you have a pain or symptom, you go to the doctor, they do tests, they figure out what is wrong, they give you medication or treatment, and you get better - but I learned that when it's chronic, it does not happen that way. There are ups and downs, and everything in between.

For a long time in the beginning, things were hard for me to digest, and being around him when things were bad was very taxing on me. Being around someone a lot that is constantly suffering and in pain, was not good for my mental health, and it was something that took some serious contemplating and self awareness to try and fix. One thing that was devastatingly hard to come to terms with was that no matter how hard I wanted to try and take his pain away, I could not. For a long time, I would stress myself out with his symptoms and how he was feeling. It was hard not to let what he went through affect me, and it was even harder to talk about. There was a long period of time where I felt depressed and had bad anxiety because there was nothing that I could do to ease anything he was going through. It was hard for me to stand by and watch someone I cared about so much be in so much pain, and struggle, and not be able to give anything other than moral support. I became angry and upset at what he had to go through, which put even more strain on my mental health.

I tried to hide this from him because I did not want him to worry or stress out about me when he had his own shit to deal with. I felt that anything I was going through was exceedingly undermined by everything he had been through and continued to go through, and that it was not worth mentioning because he had bigger fish to fry.

I, as well, constantly felt guilty that I was able to go out, be limitless in terms of my capabilities, and what I could do, when Ryan was struggling just to be able to do simple tasks. I felt guilty going out and having fun. I felt guilty hanging out with my friends and going on adventures with them, because I knew many of Ryan's friends had seemingly abandoned him when times got hard. Going out was something that I started to dread because in the back of my head I knew that he was at home, in pain, and it would just break my heart. I always wanted to be there for him and take his mind off everything.

However, Ryan was never one to guilt trip or make me feel bad for enjoying my life, quite the opposite in fact. He encouraged me, and at times forced me to go out and have fun, and to stop worrying about him. It took me quite some time to be okay with this and to stop feeling guilty, but he always reminded me to take advantage of being invited out with friends, and to enjoy every little moment with them.

At some point, I came to realize that regardless of all that Ryan was going through, he was there for me as much as I was there for him, and that it was a two way street and I did not need to carry any burden. He made me realize that having pain and illness does not take away from that fact that he is still capable of handling things outside of his own situation and be my rock when I need him too. Being with someone in his situation truly does change your perspective on life, it is about taking things one day at a time and appreciating the small things. He has taught me to appreciate every opportunity that I have been given, good or bad, and to learn from them, and apply what I have learned in my everyday life. He has taught me that your health should not be taken for granted, because it can easily be taken away from you at any time. He as well taught me not to run away from my feelings, or my mental health. To tackle these issues head on, and work through them, not run away and fear them.

It has now been over 4 years since we initially met, and I can say that time has flown by, it literally feels like yesterday that we met. It has been gratifying to watch Ryan finally get answers to a lot of his symptoms, and as well, make so much progress. I have probably hung out with him more than anyone else over the last number of years, and this has given me a front row seat into how much he pushes himself to get back to a normal life. I see him work hard at his training sessions and physio. See him run his business and stay up until all hours of the night finishing art projects. Watch him meticulously write for this book which I know has become something he has worked so hard at. Watch him push himself to do more and more outings and normal activities seemingly every month, every week, and every day. We are now able to do a lot more together than we ever have before, even though I can see that he still is in a world of pain as he pushes and fights through it. As gratifying as this progress is, I always try to keep a level head, because like many people with chronic pain and illness, there are setbacks and flair ups, where for days or weeks he will be incapacitated again. But we both have learned how to deal with these hard times, and even if I am struggling with it, seeing him be optimistic and positive through it all lets me know not to fret and worry. He always seems to smile and laugh no matter what and come out  the other side stronger.

My time with Ryan has been a gift and I continue to cherish every single moment I spend with him to the fullest. Regardless of how hard it may be sometimes, Ryan has changed my life in so many ways for the better, and I can confidently say that I am a better person since meeting him."

# Chapter 23:

## Perspective "C"

"I have loved Ryan for fourteen years. It started in a mixed grade legal studies class, where a seventeen-year-old boy caught the eye of a fifteen-year-old me, and the rest, as they say, was history. I will admit that I was immediately smitten. An older boy, sweet, funny, and devastatingly cute, looked at me, in that way that people who want to be seen crave. I had only dreams of dating, but I could never have been prepared for the friendship that would come from my crush.

As we grew closer in class, we discovered that we worked at the same local grocery store, in different sections; he, in produce, I, in customer service. There we exploited the internal telephone lines to alleviate our grocery induced boredom. Parties, New Years, bowling, restaurant hunting, and movies would be our regular activities. When the sun went down, he often would sneak into my window where we would watch movies and gossip.

As we got older, reaching legal age, our adventures became a bit wilder and our bond closer. It would be in the early hours of the morning that we would find ourselves still talking about ourselves in ways that we had never shared with anyone else.

We confided in one another, about our fears, our secrets- the darkest and ugliest parts of ourselves that we hid from everyone else. Ryan has always been this person to whom I could have the upmost faith in, trusting him with not only my real self, but someone to whom I could aspire to be. That is why this has been so devastating.

Watching someone you love become a ghost of who they are- fogged by pain and shackled by something unknown and debilitating, is heartbreaking. Here was my friend, the guy who worked out and ate protein bars, within grasping distance of his schooling being done and his career being launched; unable to get out of bed. How do you comfort someone that was just coming into his own, only to have it snatched away? I still do not know how to answer that.

I remember when it first started happening. He hid it from me in the only way he knew how, by avoiding me. Ryan has always been the type to hide his pain- from those he loves to not burden them; and from others to not appear weak. I had not heard from or seen him in a while, but he had just started his internship and I had recently entered a relationship, so life seemed like a normal excuse for his sudden absence from my life. How was I to know?

He asked me to go for dinner, at a fusion Vietnamese place that we had dined at before. I eagerly said yes, only thinking of the mouth-watering dish that I had eaten last time, I was completely unprepared for the news he had to share. He picked me up, and I did not notice right away, too excited to be finally together after so long apart. Thinking back, the silent car ride should have told me something was amiss. After we were seated, and our orders had been taken, he let me know that he had something important to tell me. I could feel the air shift just then, and I finally really looked at him. His face told me something was wrong as he struggled to find the words. Suddenly, I remembered all the times he had mentioned within the last year of him having migraines and vertigo, and I began to fear the worst. 'Oh God, does he have a brain tumour?' Knowing me as well as I knew him, he seemingly read my mind, and said that the symptoms he was having were getting much worse and were frightening and overwhelming. He feared something was very wrong, like cancer, but that he was going for tests to rule it out.

Reaching across the table, I held his hand, and I cried a little, before I tried to crack some stupid joke that escapes me now. He laughed in that way that only Ryan can, even as he was fighting against the pain that was slowly taking over his life. We carried on dinner afterwards as if all was well, but when we got back to my place, I held onto him for a long while, afraid he would disappear the moment I let him go; a strange feeling, that's for sure.

It is strange to wonder if a concrete diagnosis like cancer would have been an easier outcome than the constant tests and unconfirmed diagnosis and dozens of prescriptions that would follow instead. The years that followed were hard for him to endure, and it made me angry that something so awful could happen to someone so kind. It was not just the pain and the endless tunnels of doctors and medicine, but the disbelief he encountered from people that was equally hard to see. It is one thing to not have a doctor believe you, but when it is someone you care about, like friends - that was perhaps one of the more demoralizing aspects to witness. I am still incredibly bitter towards several people because of how they treated him. I recognize that his illness is one that is unseen, and therefore it is hard for people to understand, especially when there are no tangible answers. But then, how could they see Ryan, a man who had spent years doing the best at everything he put his mind to, suddenly throw it all away for something imaginary? I struggle to understand the lack of trust and empathy towards someone such as he.

To get his mind off the suffering, Ryan and I spent many nights battling it out on Mario Kart and fiercely competing for stars in Mario Party. I obviously won most of the time- I could not very well let his illness become a point of pity. Obviously. But sometimes, he would come over and just lie in my bed and cry. I would lie there next to him quietly, and just be there for him, even though I could do nothing to ease his pain. Those were the hardest moments, seeing him hurt and being powerless to help him.

During all of this, my life kept moving forward, and he tried his best to be a part of important events. When my now husband and I got engaged, I remember maintaining a level of hopefulness during the planning stages, thinking maybe *this* treatment he was on would be enough, *this* diagnosis would be the correct one and the one to set him on a path of recovery. So badly I wanted Ryan there on my big day that I allowed myself to believe that this disease was not as lasting as it had been thus far. As it was, he could not attend my wedding in the Dominican Republic, as the flight would have been too much. Having to walk the aisle without my best friend there alongside me was difficult and upsetting to say the least. The feeling of disappointment and frustration nagged at the edges of my mind. Why was life so unfair? The rational part of me knew this was not happening to *me,* but I could not stave off how personal this felt. It began to seem as though I was being punished through him.

After the wedding, I began to see him less and less; his days being swallowed by appointments and suffering. He was trapped in a cycle of trials and fleeting alleviation that always found him back in pain. I had to distance myself emotionally at this point, though I never stopped offering support. I was not angry at *him*, but rather at this invisible force that had stolen my friend and replaced him with a broken changeling. No longer could we spend hours binge watching crime dramas or gallivanting across the city in search of new food spots. Gone were the days of ease and fun. It was always a gamble of whether he would even be up to see me, let alone was I able to entertain the idea of living up ours 20s as we had always planned. Because he has always been 'my person', the one constant friendship that I had, I was left feeling isolated and forgotten. I think that happens often to people who are close with those with chronic pain. A part of you becomes trapped with them, strangled by your love for them, taunted by the moving goal posts that marked his return to who he was.

With the arrival of my daughter, he pushed it all to the side so that he could spend as many good days as he had holding her and making her laugh. We would go for lunch, people would congratulate him as he held her, and he never wanted to correct anyone about her parentage. At times such as these, it was easy to forget all that he was going through. Fleeting moments of his true self that he desperately pushed to the surface would mask the reality. His joy, while real, was almost always forced. It took but a look into heavy laden eyes to tell the storm that raged within, the battle that he was constantly undertaking.

It was around this time that he began to paint. It began as a method of catharsis, teaching himself how to create with water colours. I am the proud owner of some of his earliest work, including some first attempts at faces. But my most cherished piece is the one he did of my baby and dog, in a bed of fallen leaves. The way in which he would capture small parts of those he painted, forever frozen in beautiful moments, was truly a talent to behold.  I had never thought of Ryan as an artist type before he got sick, so to see what he was capable of while dealing with so much was surprising. As but a spectator to his struggle, it was like seeing the proverbial silver lining on the greyest of clouds.

With his recent diagnosis of Lyme Disease, I once again saw a glimmer of hope. Finally! Answers! But those answers were so much more complicated than I knew. Because Canadian testing for Lyme Disease is outdated and flawed, people that have lived undiagnosed with it for years suffer long term damage, and false negatives are a normal occurrence. It is maddening to know what is wrong, and for our medical system to fail him yet again. Further treatment could mean expensive bills, or even leaving for Europe, and a bill that should be covered is now hanging over his head. It made me lose faith in our healthcare, which I had always before held to such high esteem. How could a system I had revered so, be failing my friend this badly?

Watching his struggle has made me learn a lot about what kind of person he is. I always knew Ryan was kind, smart and dedicated, he showed that time and time again at work, at school and in our friendship- but this made me learn he was strong, stronger than anyone I know. His perseverance and unwillingness to give up, no matter how dark things get, has been one of the greatest inspirations to me. His determination to get the most out of life, to get back up after getting pushed down over and over, has given me strength when he did not even know it. I am deeply humbled by the kind of man he is, and eternally grateful for the role he has played in my life. Even sick, Ryan has been the most reliable and truest of friends, and I am lucky to have chanced upon his friendship all those years ago. It is my wish that his name will lend strength to my son, who will bare Ryan as his middle name.

At the end of this, I do not know if I will ever get back the person that was there so many years ago. After almost a decade of chronic pain, can anyone be who they were before? When so much time has passed, can any of us claim to be who we once were? I am unsure if I will ever get answers for my questions. And I think I am still learning to be okay with that. I miss what we had, though nothing has really diminished in that capacity. I still love Ryan as much now, if not more, than I did before all this began. I still cherish our moments together, even if they are few and far between. I still know that he is 'my person', and that our friendship is one that will endure.

I know now that life is so much more unpredictable than we know. Every moment that we get to share with those we love is precious and exceedingly hard to come by. Having a best friend that has chronic pain has taught me levels of patience and acceptance that I never knew possible. It has strengthened my compassion and empathy, to where I constantly question what goes on behind the curtain for everyone now. Seeing how easily people dismissed Ryan, it made me realize how quick people are to believe the worst in others instead of leaning into their love. In all of this, I found beauty amongst the pain, but I also witnessed the putrid rot that people carry around inside them. I sincerely hope that his story will help shed light on the hidden illnesses that so many people live with, and will teach people that we really don't know what lays beyond the masks people wear to simply survive."

# Part 4: Questions and answers!

## Chapter 24: Q&A

I thought I would end off the book by doing sort of a question and answer segment. Over the years I have done a few Q&A sessions on social media, and as well receive a ton of questions in my mailbox. I have pulled some of these to include in this segment to hopefully fill in any gaps I may have missed and tie up any sort of loose ends. Or hey, maybe you just wanted to get to know me better! So here they are!

**I have chronic pain and constantly feel guilty and have regrets about things, do you?**

I think it is just natural to feel guilty and have regrets about a lot of things, especially if you are dealing with chronic pain and illness. There is going to be a lot of guilt tied in with family or friends. Whether that is feeling like you are a burden, feeling like you need a lot of help from them, feeling like they are giving more to you, than you can give back to them. As well, there is the other side of the spectrum where you feel bad that you can't hang out with your friends or family as much as you'd like to, feeling bad that you are sometimes limited in what you can do when you can see them, and probably loads more that I am missing.

There can also be regrets about yourself, like perhaps you feel you should have caught on to your symptoms faster, taken them more seriously at the beginning, had received different opinions from doctors, said different things during different appointments, tried harder to find answers, or thought you could have prevented things all together.

In the beginning, yes, I felt a lot of these things above, and it made me feel so much worse about my situation, and about myself. I was constantly second guessing myself, blaming myself, and just feeling bad for having my family and friends be along with me for this journey. I saw how badly people were hurting when I was hurting. How can you not feel bad about that?

But over time, I learned I cannot put that amount of burden on myself. I had to really remember that I did not wish this upon myself, I did not choose to have these things happen to me, and there are some things that I just cannot help. I was almost more worried about those around me, than myself. I realized that the best thing I could do was just to focus on getting better, focus on putting in the work needed to survive this pain and illness, and focus on doing what I can to provide for myself and be independent. I look at every day as a learning experience and instead of regretting something, looking to see how I can learn from that experience and grow as a person.

**What is the hardest thing about living with chronic pain?**

Is "everything" an appropriate answer, haha. I don't know that there is just one thing that is the hardest, but one thing that is hard is knowing that when you go to sleep, you will wake up tomorrow and have to deal with all the pain and symptoms all over again. But one thing I learned that is if I put in an honest day's work of doing all the things I need to do to try and feel better, if I pushed myself outside of my comfort zone, if I accomplished something meaningful that day, even as something as simple as putting a smile on someone's face, than it makes it a lot easier to lay my head on the pillow. Knowing that I can still accomplish so much, while being so limited, keeps me thinking of the positive, and not the negative.

Another hard thing is just the unpredictability. The fact that one day symptoms can be manageable and I can go out and almost do anything, and the next day, things be so bad that I am crying in bed all day, really can take its' toll on you. It makes it impossible to plan anything. It makes you wonder why you cannot have good days all the time. It makes you question if you did something to trigger the pain and symptoms. This unpredictability also pertains to the future. Where I do not know how long I will be living with this. Will things get better? Will I be able to do all the things I wanted to do in my life? What will the next day bring? Like I mentioned in the previous section, focusing on the present moment, the present day, is all

I can do, and is all I have control over. I just must take what a certain day gives me and make the most out of it.

**How do you seem to keep so resilient through everything?**

I try to be open and honest about my journey, both in person, and social media. There are many posts where I write about how hard things are. No one sees the countless days where I cry or cannot get out of bed. I think this is true for just about anyone with chronic pain/illness. Not many people see the absolute worst, usually only a select few close family or friends.

So I do have hard days and hard times, and don't try to hide that fact, so even though it may seem at times like I'm superman or something for dealing with all this, I am still ,in fact, human haha. There are people dealing with much worse. But, again, I think many of us with chronic pain/illness are resilient, because we have to be our whole life is usually simplified down to just "surviving". For me, I just try to utilize all the tools outlined in the second part of the book. Always try to remain positive, laugh, push myself, and grow. The days I feel good, I value so much, and never take them for granted.

**How much financial burden has there been for you dealing with chronic pain/illness?**

I will not get into specific numbers, but a lot. Like I mentioned in my story, all this started when I was 22--23, finishing school, and just making my way out into the world and being independent. I was looking forward to starting my career, moving out, travelling, and exploring. As mentioned earlier, I was able to work part-time for the first couple years but have not been able to work at a job since 2015, other than a few shifts when I tried to go back in 2019. Having my own art business has helped, but I do not make near enough to support myself.  Along with not working, you add onto that there is the actual cost of treatments, and medications, and just the cost of living. I do not think the average person realizes just how much you spend just trying to get better or alleviate symptoms.

For me, I do not have any savings. Every month whatever I make goes to pay for treatment, or just living expenses. Because of this I obviously must rely on my parents for everything else.

Money, unfortunately, is one of the things that I stress about. If I do not get a lot of commissions in a certain month, it can really hamper me financially. As well, there is the guilt of, at 30 years old, having your parents still have to look after me somewhat. They should be using that money that they spent their whole lives saving for, on themselves, not me.

**Do you feel sometimes that you are worthless because of not being able to work a regular job?**

For awhile yes. But overtime I realized that I am more than my job, or my work. My value does not have to come from that. Having a career in the criminal justice field is something that I want, that I am passionate about, and that I have my degree in. But, since I am not able to work a job at the moment, I must find other ways to find self worth. For me, this includes being an advocate for the chronic pain and illness community, raising awareness, and helping those who reach out to me. Anytime that I can give back and share what I have gone through and learned, and maybe help someone, it is very important to me. Art is another way I can feel self worth, where I can make something meaningful for someone.

Most people, I believe, feel the most self worth from their job or career. It can take up most of your time and your life, so it is only natural. But when you cannot work anymore, there is a void. Everybody is different, but there are lots of ways to fill this void, and not feel like you are worthless. We spend so much of our lives keeping "busy" that we do not get to fully explore who we are, and what we find self worth in doing.

**What got you interested in studying criminal justice, and do you think it helped you in anyway with your journey? Do you think you will get into this field once you are better?**

I had a hard time after high school figuring out what I wanted to do for the rest of my life, and an equally as hard time on what to study in university. Even after I took a year off to try to figure things out, I was not sure. Initially I was in television and radio broadcasting, but I soon realized that I did not feel passionate about it, and I was not engaged at all with the content. I then switched to sport and rec business and entrepreneurship, but this was almost worse. I realized right away it was not the program for me.

I will have to thank my friend Trevor for getting me interested in criminal justice. I remember he was in first year, and I saw a few things that he was working on, and it was interesting. It was between social work and criminal justice, both of which I got into, but ultimately decided on the latter, and I am happy I made that decision.

As mentioned earlier, I was not the best student early on, and I think many in first year, found the transition to university life hard. A turning point came after a professor wrote this message on the back of my final paper. "In class you present as distant, unattached to anything, and free to come and go as you please. To learn about yourself one has to be prepared to interact with others. This is not something you cherish so you choose to sit alone at the back of the room. You present as pleasant, easy going and harmless. If you are not in class, few would notice, and this is a hell of an indictment to put on any human being. You have 3 years to change the above, it's time to get serious to start being assertive and to leave your mark on those you encounter."

At the time, this comment greatly angered me. I had just finished writing a paper entitled, Who Am I? in which we were supposed to write about how we became the person we are today. A lot of my paper was me opening up about the bullying I experienced, and how that shaped me. And how at 19 years old, it was still impacting me. I wrote about my struggles talking and opening up to people, because at that time I still feared being made fun of. At this time, I had not learned to love myself, be proud of myself, or like who I was. I thought he would be more empathetic reading about my struggles, but in his comment, it almost seemed the opposite.

It was not until I realized that this teacher was just trying to motivate me, when I switched from being mad at his message, to understanding. I was still very young, but I needed to put more work both into myself, and university. I needed to stop coasting by. I needed to live up to my potential. So, thanks to that message, it put me on the right path, I just wish he maybe would have talked to me in person, instead of writing a note.

In school, interestingly, there were classes in which we studied addiction, and got into the rehabilitation methods that were used when someone is trying to break their habit. There is a lot of similarities between methods or coping skills of dealing with chronic pain, and methods or coping skills of dealing with addiction. I believe this prior knowledge came in handy since I was very familiar with the skills and terminology when faced with pain years later.

It is this area, addictions, that I would like to get into if I ever get back into the field, or helping others overcome difficulties, as I feel like I have a lot to offer. Although I do not have any experience in being an addict, or criminal etc.  I do have experience in many areas in which I think I could pass along and help someone.

**How do you deal with people or friends that do not seem to care or understand what you go through? Or those that make rude comments.**

Unfortunately, when you speak out as much as I do about the subject, there are bound to be a few outspoken individuals who will openly question you. I have heard everything. From saying that I am faking, looking for attention, exaggerating, a snowflake, and questioning if any of what I go through is even real. It has happened mostly online, but in person as well, but more behind my back than to my face. I think the majority of those with chronic issues have heard similar things as well, and it is heartbreaking to see. All I can do is be open and honest about my journey, answer questions if anybody has any, and then it is out of my control what people think of me. To a normal person they just are not going to understand what I feel and go through. And the truth is, they are not going to understand, unless they have gone through something similar themselves. Or even have a loved one go through something similar. It is frustrating, but that is the reality. They just are never going to know what it is like; it is something that you must experience. I think people do not fully understand how impairing chronic pain/illness can be, and how it literally impacts everything. I think it is sad when people make crude comments. but I cannot stop them. If it is someone that I do not know, I just must ignore it. I cannot make everyone happy, and I cannot make everyone believe me. I cannot waste my time and energy on someone, especially if they do not want to learn and educate themselves. A lot of time, hurting someone, or "trolling" is their only goal.

The harder part is when it is a friend or family member who does not care what I am going through, or questions it. Friends and family are very important to me, and I always try to make my them feel important and loved. But, if I do not get that in return, it is one of the worst feelings. I have had many people who I thought would be lifelong friends, turn their back on me when times got hard. Friends who showed no empathy, no caring, and did not even try to be there for me. All I can do in this situation is just realize that they may not be the people that I thought they were, and if it is necessary, just remove them from social media and my life. I cannot force people to want to be friends with me, and I cannot force them to go through this journey with me. But what this journey has done is make me realize how special the people in my life are, that have stuck by me.

**What is something simple, or free, that a person can do by themselves to help with pain?**

One that I think is very important but often overlooked is myofacial release. Or more simply, self massage. Many people, no matter if they are in pain or not, will have multiple areas on their body that are tense, that have knots, and that are tender. Overtime, if not addressed, these knots can grow bigger, become painful, and even affect nerves and your range of motion.

Instead of paying $100 dollars an hour for a massage, doing simple research, or watching YouTube videos on myofacial release, can be just as beneficial. There are many cheap tools and equipment that can aid in this process. If you want to spend a bit of money, massage guns can help a lot, although they will not get deep into some muscles like you may need.

The second thing is breathing exercises. After I got diagnosed with a breathing disorder, I did a ton of research on the subject, and read many books. It greatly surprised me that 90% of us are breathing incorrectly, or not optimally. And this makes sense as it is something that we really never think about. But how come so many of us are breathing so bad? A lot of it comes down to stress levels.

Breathing abnormally can impact such a large number of functions in our body. It can make you feel sick, dizzy, cause muscle tension, fatigue, worsening anxiety, and depression, limit our physical capabilities like exercise, and if you have any underlying health issues, make those symptoms worse.

The road to breathing correctly is not a hard one, and something you can do on your own, although it can take awhile for your body to adjust and to feel benefits. One of the easiest things is just to be more mindful during the day about your breathing. Do I hold my breath a lot? Do I breathe through my nostrils all the time? (correct), or do I sometimes breathe in through my mouth (incorrect). When I breathe in, does my diaphragm expand? (correct). Or does only one of my chest/belly expand? (incorrect) When I exhale, does my tummy contract? (correct).

Googling breathing exercises and implementing them in your everyday life can be beneficial. And it can take as little as 5 minutes a day. Other things like meditation, exercise, and yoga can also help.

A device I use is called the emwave2. This hooks up to your ear lobe, and to the computer, and measures your heart rate and your breathing pattern, and offers many different types of exercises. Its nice to see in real time the impact that a correct breathing pattern can have, and for me I have found a reduction in pain levels.

**How has chronic pain/illness affected your ability to have a romantic relationship?**

I am totally open and honest about myself, and about my journey, but what I do keep private is anything about my family or my relationships, especially online. But I can answer the question while maintaining the privacy of others.

For the first many years of my journey, I did not even entertain the idea of a relationship. I did not even go out on a date, or kiss anyone. My symptoms were so bad, that it was just something that was impossible. It would have been both unfair to me, and a potential partner, to seek any sort of relationship at that time. I was always comfortable being single, and never one to really care if I was in a relationship or not, so it did not bother me. At this time, I just really needed to focus on myself.

About halfway through my journey, I made the decision to be more open about the possibility of dating. Even though my symptoms were still overwhelming, I figured if I was open and honest about what I was going through, a potential partner could make their own decision whether to pursue anything with me.

I quickly learned though that a normal relationship was almost impossible to have. I was so limited in what I could do. So many dates I had, were super simple, such as just getting coffee, or going for a small walk or drive. For many years, very simple dates like this was all I could do. I will not dive in too much more than that, but I will just say that I admire anyone who is in a relationship with someone in chronic pain or has a chronic illness. You often must give so much of yourself and be so selfless. You ride the waves of the ups and downs with that person, and that can be exhausting. You must compromise so much. But, from experience, having a strong, loving, and healthy relationship is possible while dealing with chronic issues.

**If I am feeling down on a particular day, is there a quick mental exercise you recommend?**

Something that is quick and easy, is to write down things that you are grateful for, sort of like a gratification journal. From what I have learned, it is helpful to write what you are grateful for and divide it into three sub sections, people/pets you are grateful for, something about yourself that you like and are grateful for, and something you are grateful for about the world. Expanding on these into a small paragraph on each, and reading them over can reaffirm just how lucky you are, and that even if you are having a bad day, there are things to smile and be happy about. Sometimes we need a gentle reminder.

If I were to do an entry for myself, it may look like this: I am grateful for my dog Finn. Everyday when I get home, he greets me with overwhelming joy, leaping into my chest, and a bark that is indistinguishable. Different from his usual barks. This makes me feel loved and that he cares about me, as much as I care about him. I am grateful for his company in the hardest of moments, and his nonstop need to follow me wherever I go. He makes me laugh and smile all the time, especially when he sleeps, as he flips on his back, legs sprawled out, mouth half open.

I am grateful for my sense of humor. It does not matter how I feel, it seems as though I can always appreciate a good joke or am on the lookout to tell a funny one myself. Laughing myself, or seeing others laugh is truly like a medicine, it makes me feel better, and for a few fleeting moments, I forget everything for just a few seconds.

I am grateful to be surrounded by such scenery and nature as I am. It takes only a 2-minute walk, and I am down by the river, surrounded by endless trees, shrubs, animals, and birds. It is nice to get away from the concrete jungle for awhile, and just explore, listen to the sounds of nature, and let my senses guide my train of thought. It makes me happy that I can enjoy this either by myself, or with my friends and family.

An entry would be as simple as that, it took me about 5 minutes. A few short paragraphs, going into a bit of detail on each. You might notice that while writing it out, you may crack a smile, feel a sense of calm, or a sense of appreciation. Positive memories and visuals may come to mind. I do not think there is a limit as to how often to practice an exercise like this. Once a day, once a week, or whenever you feel like it. However, if you are making it a regular occurrence, I think it would be best to try to write on a new thing that you are grateful for, then the previous entry.

**It seems throughout your journey you have had a tough time with doctors. Do you hold any anger or resentment towards them?**

I think it would be easy for me to point the finger and lay blame elsewhere, specifically towards doctors for not taking me seriously, giving me wrong advice, not digging deeper to find the root cause etc. But at the end of the day, they are human too. And while yes, I have been frustrated numerous times over the years, I do not hold any anger or hostility.

In terms of family doctors, their scope of what they must know about is so broad. They basically must know a little about everything. Whereas, if you are a specialist, your work revolves around a specific area. So, when something is complex, rarely seen, or different, it is rare for a family doctor to know right away what is going on. For example, my latest family doctor said he has only ever had one other patient with Lyme. With that rarity, Lyme is not going to be on his radar, or something he thinks about that often. Family doctors in my experience, are usually pretty good at referring elsewhere to a specialist if it is something they feel needs to be looked at.

A problem I also noticed is that doctors are often over worked, and constantly busy. I have been to enough doctors' offices and appointments over the years to notice that they are always running behind. This often leads to appointments feeling rushed or feeling like they are trying to get you out of the door as quickly as possible. Instead of intently listening to a patient, and their concerns, their mind seems to be on other things. I think if the medical system was less busy, and doctors had more opportunities to spend quality time with their patients, less things would be missed, and there would be a stronger doctor patient relationship, which I have learned is very important.

I have also noticed that some push medications quite hard, thinking that they are the only answer. While medications may help alleviate symptoms, they often do not cure whatever is ailing the patient. I always became frustrated at doctors wanting to treat my symptoms, but them not diving into more of the root problem, or why I was having these symptoms. I was also frustrated as it seems most doctors will never admit if they do not know what is going on. Usually in this case, they place the blame on the patient, saying it is anxiety, depression, or in that realm. In the end, I have the utmost respect for doctors, and most of them are trying their best, and want the best for their patients. But even so, the human body is so complex that it is impossible to assume they have all the answers. That is why, as I have written before, it is important that we do our own research, get educated, and get as many different opinions as we feel we need.

**What is one thing that people often overlook when they see someone dealing with chronic pain/illness?**

I would say the mental side. This even gets overlooked by those suffering as well. For many people, when they have pain, it is for a short duration, and they know when it is going to heal or subside. But, with chronic pain/illness, it is always there. Often, we do not know when it is going to subside, if ever. This constant pain or symptoms eventually takes its' toll. You wake up, it is there. You go outside, it is there. You try to do any activities, it is there. Overtime, it can lead to a loss of sleep, loss of appetite, loss of function, loss of friends, loss of job, loss of purpose. There can be a lot of loss. When you combine this with people not taking you seriously, making fun of you, doctors brushing you off, it is a recipe for a mental disaster.

When I mean that the mental side often gets overlooked by those suffering as well, I mean that we often neglect or do not realize how seriously we need to be taking care of our mental health. Like I mentioned during my journey, for the first few years, I hardly did anything to look after myself mentally. I always had the mentality that things would just eventually go away and get better. I was not prepared for this to be long lasting, and I did not have any sort of coping skills when things really got bad. The big reason I wrote the second part of the book, on how I mentally dealt with my chronic issues, was because it was one of the most important steps that I took for myself, and it helped me immensely. I know if I neglected my mental health, then maybe others who are suffering like me are too. It was a big motivating factor to write this book.

**I have a few friends that suffer from chronic illness and pain. What can I do to help?**

From writing about my experiences and my journey, I have had many people contact me that they have a friend or loved one who is dealing with chronic issues, and what can they do to help, and how can they be a better friend, better father, brother etc. As you can imagine there is no short answer to this question, and every case will be different, so I can only answer this question from personal experience. From my perspective, I did not want to be defined by what afflicted me; I did not want my relationship with others to be all about me and my pain. In my day to day relationships, I want to be seen as the person I am, and treated normally, like everyone else. What helped was a friend or loved one just being there with me. Doing things such as playing board games, going for walks, going out for a coffee, or running errands; simple things. Activities that are relaxing, where we can have a laugh, and have a conversation. If I were having a good day, I wanted someone who would push my boundaries and suggest doing things that I have not been able to do for a while. If I was having a bad day, I wanted it to be okay if all we did was relax, watch TV, or play video games. I wanted to be surrounded by people that were positive, that had an optimistic view of the world. I wanted to be surrounded by people that were laid back, that told jokes and did not take things too seriously. I think it is also important for a friend or family member of someone dealing with chronic pain or illness to give compliments and point out any progress that you may see. Give affection like a hug or a kiss, or any sort of gesture that shows you care.

I think many people have an idea in their head that all we want to talk about is our issues, or how hard we have it, and use others as a literal punching bag to get things off our chest, or to vent, rant, and complain. From having met others who have chronic issues, I can see where this idea may come from, as some people make it the focal point of their conversations with others. Some people do not have the awareness about how much they talk about their issues. If you have a friend like this, the best thing you can do is just listen, but eventually try to steer the conversation away to something else. Try to do activities with them that may distract them. As I mentioned in the previous chapters, you do not want your relationship with your friend to be all about them and their issues.

You may also have friends who are the opposite and never talk about what they are going through and that may become distant, where you do not see them or talk to them for a while. It is very common for those suffering to have anxiety, depression, or even embarrassment about their situation where they withdraw from relationships. I had periods where I felt like a burden to people, that I did not want to waste their time, and where I didn't want people to see me at my worst, and so vulnerable. Those with chronic issues know what we deal with affects our relationships with others, and we know that it can be hard to be with someone who is in distress. During some of my most difficult moments I saw firsthand, those suffering along with me, and it made me feel so bad and so guilty.  If you have a friend of loved one who is showing signs of withdrawing, the best thing you can do is show that you care, and that you are interested, by being the one to make contact with them,  asking how they are doing, asking what is new, and if everything is okay. As well, making an effort in asking them to hangout, all the while being mindful in what their limitations may be, and that they may say no.

The best qualities that you as a friend or loved one can have are patience, and empathy. A lot of days we may be a mess, we might not be able to hangout, we might get easily angered and our emotions may be all over the place. Sometimes we may even lash out and take out our anger or frustrations on you. But it is not personal, and it is nothing that you did or said, and it is not your fault. Chronic issues take its toll mentally, and it is unfortunate that those closest to us may get the brunt of it. It is natural for someone to want to back away from this situation, to desensitize themselves, or to completely abandon the relationship; it can be a strain and it is not easy. But I urge you to fight it out. Having chronic issues can be the loneliest feeling in the world, and in my case, having friends and loved ones stick by me and support me, meant everything.

# Chapter 25:

## The End

This brings us to the end of J.R.R. Tolkens saga, Lord of the Rings. I thank you from the bottom of my heart for taking the time to read about my journey, what I have learned, and everything in between. It is my hope that perhaps you have learned something, or in the very least, saw life from a different perspective. I will certainly miss writing, editing, and coming up with random thoughts to put into this book at all hours of the night. I will miss the days I could not see straight and used a talk to text application to garner thoughts and ideas, to write out at a later date when I felt better. I will miss the gratifying feeling of writing one more page, one more word.

If you are reading this, and are going through chronic issues yourself, just know that you are strong. Stronger than you think you know. There are people that are so proud of you; I am proud of you. We have been dealt a bad hand, but it is how we play this hand that ultimately matters. No matter where you are in your journey right now, just remember how far you have come, and remember to put in the work to get even farther. We are still capable of achieving great things, still capable of happiness, still capable of feeling peace.

If you are not going through chronic issues, the message honestly does not change. Just because you are not going through chronic health issues, does not mean that you might be going through something else, or have in the past. We all have ups and downs; we all have challenges. So, it is the same message. You are also stronger than you think you are. You, as well, have people that are proud of you. As well, remember how far you have come, and likewise, put in the work to get even farther.

Over the years, I have come to accept the fate that has happened to me. Come to accept the struggle, the ups and downs, and the lingering uncertainty of the future. I spent so many years resisting, pushing back, and wishing so badly for my life to go back to the way it was. As I wrote, this only made things worse, and harder. This experience has forever changed me, but I choose to look at this change in a good way. I choose to embrace the experiences I went through, learn from them, and come out the other side as wise as I can be, Gandalf level wise! Accepting my fate does not mean that I give up, quite the opposite in fact. I am accepting what has happened to me but working as hard as I can to make the most out of my situation. Learning what I can do to make the most out of my life, with the limitations I have been given. I do not know what the future holds for me, but I sure am going to work my butt off to find out.

I encourage all of you to strive to be the best versions of yourself. Stay true to who you are. You are your own unique person, and personality. Do not be afraid to show it. Do not be afraid to have opinions, and fight for what you believe in. Do not be afraid to speak up. Do not be afraid to learn, grow, and make mistakes along the way. Do not be afraid to love and show love. As a special friend once told me, "Life has no smooth road for any of us. As we go down it, we need to remember that happiness is a talent we develop, not an object we seek. It is the ability to bounce back from life's inevitable setbacks. Some people are crushed by misfortune, others grow because of it."

If you have enjoyed reading, feel free to pass this book along, or recommend it to someone else! I am always available to get a hold of, for whatever reason. Questions, comments, concerns, queries, knock knock jokes. You name it. As well, you can contact me if you would like the contact information of any of the practitioners that were featured. My email is **ry.artwork55@gmail.com**. My instagram is **ry_artwork**. My website is **www.ryartwork.com**. My home address is wherever you want me to be. Thank you for reading.

www.ingramcontent.com/pod-product-compliance
Lightning Source LLC
Chambersburg PA
CBHW051442250726
48655CB00001B/196